Nutrition in the '90s

Current Controversies and Analysis

edited by
Gerald E. Gaull
Frank N. Kotsonis
Maureen A. Mackey

The NutraSweet Company
Deerfield, Illinois

Marcel Dekker, Inc. New York · Basel · Hong Kong

Library of Congress Cataloging-in-Publication Data

Nutrition in the '90s : current controversies and analysis / edited by
Gerald E. Gaull, Frank N. Kotsonis, Maureen A. Mackey.
p. cm.
Includes bibliographical references and index.
ISBN 0-8247-8525-8
1. Nutrition--Congresses. I. Gaull, Gerald E. II. Kotsonis,
Frank N. III. Mackey, Maureen A.
QP141.A1N8657 1990
613.2--dc20 90-23846
CIP

This book is printed on acid-free paper.

Marcel Dekker, Inc.
270 Madison Avenue, New York, New York 10016

Current printing (last digit):
10 9 8 7 6 5 4 3 2

PRINTED IN THE UNITED STATES OF AMERICA

Preface

The 1980s was a decade of public policy decisions in the field of nutrition. The Department of Health and Human Services and the Department of Agriculture released their "Dietary Guidelines for Americans," seven suggestions to modify dietary and lifestyle habits to improve health. The results of the Lipid Research Clinics Coronary Primary Prevention Trials provided evidence that pharmacological reduction of blood cholesterol can reduce the risk for coronary heart disease. Thereafter, the National Heart, Lung and Blood Institute launched the National Cholesterol Education Program, and Americans started hearing about the health benefits of reducing the intake of fat and cholesterol. And toward the end of the decade, the Surgeon General and the National Research Council each issued their analyses of the relationship between diet and health. They offered dietary recommendations for Americans to control their weight, cut down on fat, particularly saturated fat, and eat more foods rich in complex carbohydrates.

The recommendations of these various organizations have given Americans a starting point from which to evaluate their individual diets and to determine the kinds of dietary changes they may want to make to improve their chances for good health. However, when attempting to put these recommendations into practice, several individual factors must be considered, including family and medical history, exercise, stress, and smoking habits. No single factor will guarantee good health and long life.

Nutritional science is a multifaceted discipline with roots in fields as diverse as epidemiology and molecular biology. Its advancement has been overshadowed in recent years by quantum leaps made in the areas of genetics, neuroscience, and molecular biology. Thus, despite the consensus among these health profession and public health organizations regarding dietary recommendations, controversy remains. This conflicting information may be confusing to the consumer. We must help the consumer understand, however, that all sciences, including nutrition, are constantly evolving, and that the database for certain issues is incomplete.

The purpose of the presentations held at The NutraSweet Company was to share with its members current information about issues in nutritional science that are still contentious and in need of further clarification. The quality and timeliness of these presentations prompted us to share them with a larger audience—thus their publication as this book. It was clear from the presentations that there are still controversies surrounding certain nutritional issues, and the new information will be useful in making decisions about diet and lifestyle. We hope the reader will better appreciate the difficulties the food industry faces in simultaneously striving to satisfy customers' demands for taste appeal and the best criteria for healthfulness in the products they produce.

Our authors come from diverse areas of nutritional science, and each is a leader in his or her field. Some dispel old nutritional myths with new evidence. For example, Dr. Jules Hirsch explains in his chapter how obesity cannot be conveniently ascribed to gluttony coupled with sloth, but rather that it most likely has its origins in genetics. Obese individuals may have a biological template that sensitizes them to such environmental influences as an overabundant food supply and a highly mechanized society. Dr. Raymond Slavin discusses the rarity of true food allergies, and defines other reactions to foods that are all too frequently self-diagnosed as "allergy." Dr. Adam Drewnowski presents evidence that the well-publicized "carbohydrate craving" experienced by obese dieters may actually be a preference for fat/sugar mixtures commonly available in foods such as chocolate, ice cream, and pastries.

Dr. Irwin Rosenberg focuses on a relatively new topic in nutritional science, i.e., the nutritional needs of our ever-growing elderly population. He points out that we do not know the nutritional requirements of people over 51 years, as evidenced by the grouping of all people 51 years and older into one category in the most recent publication of the Recommended Dietary Allowances. He cites several pieces of evidence that our elderly's needs for certain nutrients can be quite different from those of a generation younger.

Two of our contributors update us on factors that influence food intake. Dr. Susan Schiffman describes how the taste and smell of foods can be manipulated to promote food intake in the anorectic elderly, and to limit it in the dieting obese. Dr. Barbara Rolls revisits the controversy over whether food intake is controlled by internal mechanisms that sense energy balance. She indicates that, at least over the long term, normal-weight individuals may regulate their food intake to control their weight within normal limits.

Issues concerning food regulation and technology are presented by Dr. Sanford Miller and Dr. Marcus Karel. In his chapter, Dr. Miller argues that the American food industry and its regulator, the Food and Drug Administration, are facing a new challenge to develop a national policy to guide the improvement of nutritional qualities of food. As industry and academia work together to develop new technologies to produce foods that will not just alleviate hunger but will also enhance health, the FDA must adopt better ways to evaluate these products. It is obvious that cooperation among these three groups is essential if progress in these areas is to occur. Dr. Karel elaborates on some of the innovative technologies being used to develop new, more nutritious, and safer foods. Advances in food engineering and materials science will yield products with specific quality and nutritional attributes that meet the nutritional needs of population subgroups. And freshness and microbiological stability of food will be better assured by the use of new packaging materials and computer-assisted inventory control.

Dr. William Connor and Dr. Norman Kretchmer enlighten us on the relationship between certain components of our diet and health, an issue which has received much public interest lately. Dr. Connor, in Chapter 9, explains there is more to reducing one's risk for coronary heart disease than simply reducing cholesterol intake. Reduction of blood cholesterol requires modifications in intake of omega-3 and omega-6 fatty acids and complex carbohydrates, including soluble fibers. The omega-3 fatty acids offer the extra advantage of interfering with the processes that promote thrombosis, a necessary component of coronary heart disease. Dr. Kretchmer identifies the health concerns associated with typical sugar consumption as limited to dental caries. While sugar has been blamed for many other diseases or conditions, such as coronary heart disease, diabetes, and hyperactivity, there is no compelling evidence to date that sugar causes these problems.

The discussions of our contributors show us that there are a number of unresolved issues in nutritional science. These issues will demand continuing research. The 1990s present the challenge to nutritional scientists to refine and to qualify the broad generalizations of the 1980s regarding the relationship between diet and health. Additional investigations may reveal that the immense genetic diversity and environmental influences in our population will preclude the ability to make nutritional dicta appropriate for entire populations. Instead we may realize that it is necessary to segment the population and, in some cases, to take a more individualized approach to optimizing dietary recommendations.

Gerald E. Gaull
Frank N. Kotsonis
Maureen A. Mackey

Contents

About the Editors

Dr. Gerald E. Gaull has served as Vice President for Nutritional Science at The NutraSweet Company in Deerfield, Illinois, since 1984. He also holds an appointment as Adjunct Professor of Pediatrics at Northwestern University School of Medicine.

Prior to this, Dr. Gaull served as Professor of Pediatrics, Mt. Sinai School of Medicine of the City University of New York, as well as attending pediatrician at Mt. Sinai Hospital. His career in pediatrics spans some 25 years in academic research, teaching, and practice, with emphasis on nutrition, genetics, and developmental biochemistry.

Dr. Gaull graduated in 1951 from the University of Michigan and is a 1955 graduate of the Boston University School of Medicine. He is a Diplomate of the American Board of Pediatrics and is listed in *American Men and Women of Science, Who's Who in the World,* and *Who's Who in America.*

Dr. Gaull's honors include the 1978 Borden Award in nutrition and development of the American Academy of Pediatrics and the Gold Medal of St. Ambrosiano of the City of Milan (1983). He is the author of numerous published books, original communications, and articles on nutrition, genetics, and human development.

Dr. Frank N. Kotsonis is Vice President of Preclinical and Clinical Research at The NutraSweet Company, Deerfield, Illinois. He is also an Adjunct Professor of Pharmacology and Toxicology at the Philadelphia College of Pharmacy and Science. Dr. Kotsonis was director of toxicology for the Research and Development Division of G. D. Searle & Co. prior to joining The NutraSweet Company. He received his B.S. and Ph.D. (1975) degrees from the University of Wisconsin-Madison, and the M.S. degree from the University of Arizona, Tucson. He is the author of numerous articles on metabolism, nutrition, and toxicology, and is on the editorial boards of several leading scientific journals. He is also a Diplomate of the American Board of Toxicology. Dr. Kotsonis is past president of the Midwest Chapter of the Society of Toxicology and is currently on the International Life Science Institute-Nutrition Foundation Board of Trustees and the International Food Biotechnology Council Board of Directors.

Dr. Maureen A. Mackey is Associate Director of Nutritional Science at The NutraSweet Company. She received her B.S. in nutrition (1978) from the University of California, Davis, and M.S. (1981) and Ph.D. (1985) degrees from the University of Minnesota, St. Paul. Dr. Mackey has worked in the food industry for the past six years. She is also a Registered Dietitian.

About the Contributors

Dr. William E. Connor is Head of the Division of Endocrinology, Metabolism and Nutrition, Department of Medicine, Oregon Health Sciences University, Portland, Oregon. He has served as President of the American Society for Clinical Nutrition and as Editor of the *Journal of Laboratory and Clinical Medicine*. He has conducted extensive research in the area of lipids, including omega-3 fatty acids. Dr. Connor received his M.D. from the University of Iowa in 1950.

Dr. Adam Drewnowski is Associate Professor and Director, Human Nutrition Program at the University of Michigan School of Public Health, Ann Arbor. He has conducted numerous studies on the psychological aspects of abnormal eating behaviors and on the relationship between obesity and taste preferences. Dr. Drewnowski received a Ph.D. in psychology from The Rockefeller University in 1977.

Dr. Jules Hirsch serves as the Sherman Fairchild Professor and Senior Physician at The Rockefeller University and University Hospital in New York. He has a long and distinguished career in obesity research and treatment. He received the Distinguished Alumnus Award, Southwestern Medical School and The McCollum Award of the American Society for Clinical Nutrition. Dr. Hirsch received an M.D. from Southwestern Medical School, University of Texas in 1948.

Dr. Marcus Karel is Professor Emeritus, Department of Chemical Engineering, Massachusetts Institute of Technology, Cambridge Massachusetts, and Professor of Food Science at Rutgers University, New Brunswick, New Jersey. He has received numerous awards, including the Nicholas Appert Medal and the William V. Cruess Award for Excellence in Teaching, both from the Institute of Food Technologists. He holds five patents and has published extensively in the areas of physical chemistry of foods, food engineering, and food processing. Dr. Karel received a Ph.D in food technology from the Massachusetts Institute of Technology in 1960.

Dr. Norman Kretchmer is Professor, Department of Nutritional Sciences, Department of Pediatrics, and Department of Obstetrics at the University of California at Berkeley, and Director of the Koret Center for Human Nutrition, San Francisco General Hospital. He also served as Director of the National Institute of Child Health and Human Development. Dr. Kretchmer has a longstanding interest in carbohydrate metabolism and diabetes. He received a Ph.D. in physiological chemistry from the University of Minnesota in 1947 and his M.D. from the State University of New York College of Medicine in 1952.

Dr. Sanford A. Miller is Dean of the Graduate School of Biomedical Sciences and Professor, Departments of Biochemistry and Medicine, The University of Texas Health Science Center at San Antonio. He served as Director of the FDA's Center for Food Safety and Applied Nutrition from 1978 to 1987. Dr. Miller has written and spoken extensively about food safety and regulatory policy. He received his Ph.D. in physiology and biochemistry from Rutgers University in 1957.

Dr. Barbara J. Rolls is Director of the Laboratory for the Study of Human Ingestive Behavior at Johns Hopkins University, Baltimore, Maryland. She has conducted extensive research in the psychological and physiological controls of food selection and intake in man. Dr. Rolls received a Ph.D. in physiology from the University of Cambridge, England, in 1970 and spent fourteen years at the University of Oxford in England, where she conducted research on thirst and drinking.

Dr. Irwin Rosenberg is Director, USDA Human Nutrition Center on Aging, Tufts University, Boston, Massachusetts. He has served as President of the American Society for Clinical Nutrition and as Chair of the Food and Nutrition Board, National Academy of Sciences, in addition to holding numerous other offices. He is currently Editor-in-Chief of *Nutrition Reviews*. Dr. Rosenberg received his M.D. from Harvard University in 1959.

Dr. Susan S. Schiffman is Professor of Medical Psychology and Director of the Weight Loss Unit in the Department of Psychiatry at Duke University Medical Center, in Durham, North Carolina. She is an internationally recognized authority on taste and smell and their role in nutrition and human behavior. Her research spans the range from clinical to molecular investigations of the senses of taste and smell. Dr. Schiffman received a Ph.D. in psychology in 1970 from Duke University.

Dr. Raymond Slavin is Professor of Internal Medicine and Microbiology at the St. Louis University School of Medicine, Missouri. He has served as President of the American Academy of Allergy and Immunology and as President of the American Association of Immunologists. He has published extensively in the areas of immunology and allergy. He received his M.D. from St. Louis University School of Medicine in 1956.

1

Fat's Not Fun

JULES HIRSCH, M.D.[*]

Introduction

I recently learned from a local newpaper of a new depth in scientific illiteracy to which we as a nation have plunged. The comments that I read concerned a poll in which "the man in the street" was asked whether the Earth went around the sun or the sun around the Earth. Twenty-one percent of those asked had no idea which answer was correct. I know the present reader would have done better, but how well could you answer questions related to human nutrition, specifically a question about obesity? In fact, we might answer questions about nutrition less successfully than those about astronomy, because when nutrition is under consideration, everyone seems to have answers, but too often the answers are wrong.

*The Rockefeller University and University Hospital, New York, New York.

The Nature of Human Obesity

The central objective of this chapter is to dispel at least one major myth about human obesity: the idea that obesity comes about largely, if not entirely, by optional overeating, that is, a personal decision to savor the good tastes of food. A related and equally erroneous notion is that obese people elect to become physically inert simply because such behavior creates pleasant sensations. This hedonic, or pleasure-seeking, theory of obesity carries an implicit criticism of those who are obese. Obese people, it is reasoned, have somewhat selfishly made themselves what they are, thereby incurring an increased risk of illness as well as an unpleasant physical appearance. I believe this approach to human obesity is pointless and will give evidence that more basic biological factors are at work than simple personal mischief or caprice. You may remember the great 19th-century classic by Samuel Butler entitled *Erewhon*. In *Erewhon* illness is a crime, and crimes are illnesses. Someone who develops pulmonary tuberculosis deserves prolonged imprisonment, but a thief is to be treated in the most solicitous manner by expert physicians. What makes this premise so interesting and amusing is the possibility that some truth exists in what initially appears to be a preposterous proposition. I will attempt to persuade the reader that the *Erewhon* approach to obesity is neither helpful nor correct.

The most fundamental new piece of information in human biology is the recognition that there is a genetic code, a single blueprint in each organism. Four simple substances in different combinations constitute a special code in DNA that governs the production of all proteins in the human organism. It may seem surprising that such a simple code can lead to so complex a structure as man, but it is perhaps less surprising when one recognizes that the remarkable information found in a modern computer consists of a code with only two elements.

It is perhaps also surprising that so complex a system as food intake, with all its attendant environmental and psychosocial components, has major determinants in the fundamental biological code. This fact is shared by other complex systems. Thus, studies of major behavioral disorders and addictive diseases have uncovered evidence for genetic differences that create special vulnerabilities for the development of illness; nevertheless, the illness comes about only through the behaviors or interactions of the organism with the environment. In the absence of spoken words and relations with people it might be incredibly difficult or even impossible to detect schizophrenia or major depressive disorders, yet the disease is not to be found in these interactions alone, but also in the fundamental nature of the organism as it approaches these interactions. In the absence of addicting substances in the environment, there would be no discernible addiction, yet the biological structure of the organism remains a major factor in determining whether an addictive disorder will or will not occur. Likewise, in a situation of food scarcity, obesity might never occur. I will argue, however, that obesity can occur only on a certain biological template, the creation of which has preceded the abundance of food or food-related behaviors.

The Function of Fat

Obesity is best defined as an excess storage of fat in adipose tissue. The function of stored fat, other than the obvious cushioning or insulation of adipose tissue, is to serve as a source of energy that enables the intermittent intake of food. Even during the brief fast of an overnight sleep, fat is removed from adipose sites for burning in muscles and other organs. Much as an automobile can hold 5 to 10% of the weight of the vehicle as stored fuel in a full gas tank, so man carries 15% more body fat as stored energy in adipose tissue. Even the term newborn has 12 to 15% body weight as stored fat. At any stage of life, when this storage exceeds 30% the person is obese.

A more precise expression of obesity has recently found favor: the body mass index (BMI). The BMI is calculated by dividing the weight of an individual in kilograms (kg) by the square of his height in meters (m^2). Thus, BMI = kg/m^2. When this number is 27 or greater, a sufficient excess accumulation of adipose tissue exists to be a hazard to health. Such an increase in weight is roughly 20% above "ideal weight," and at least 35 million Americans suffer from this degree of obesity. The incidence of diseases such as diabetes, hypertension, and osteoarthritis, gall bladder diseases, and even some types of cancer is higher in obese people. Furthermore, accumulations of blood fat, or hyperlipidemia, often accompany obesity and can be a major risk factor for heart disease.

The central issue of obesity is why some individuals maintain a storage of fat that is fixed at a level higher than normal. Certain considerations lead one to believe that this condition must occur as a result of faulty operation of a normal regulation of stored fat. An individual of average size who weighs 70 kilograms may store 9 kilograms of fat and perhaps 10 kilograms of protein. The amount of stored carbohydrate is much less, usually not in excess of 1 kilogram. Over the course of a lifetime, however, literally tons of food and water are consumed and metabolized. The inflow and outflow are enormous compared with the small amount stored in the body. The by-products of metabolism—water, carbon dioxide, and other wastes—leave the body at a rate that assures constancy of body composition. Were there to be as little as a 1% error in the precise equality of intake and outgo, the composition of the body and its attendant stores of nutrients would either rise sharply or fall precipitously.

The fundamental and simple equation that governs intake and outgo is $\Delta E = Q - W$; that is, a change in the stored energy (ΔE) can occur only when Q, the intake of energy, exceeds W, the outgo. W is measured as a composite of work, heat, and the energy value of secreted material. Under ordinary circumstances, the caloric reserve in the form of triglyceride fats in adipose tissue is sufficient to withstand a starvation period of 30 days or more. The obese individual is uniquely endowed with the ability to withstand starvation for an even longer period, but this questionable advantage accrues only at great cost to health and physical appearance.

When one considers the terms of this equation or the metabolic "errors" that might lead to obesity, it is evident that work and heat output are not easily observed and are therefore difficult to measure. Thus, it is small wonder that great emphasis is placed on food intake—that is, the search for extra pleasure by the consumption of great amounts of food—as a primary cause of obesity. It must be pointed out, however, that the additional consumption of food required to maintain the obese state is not particularly great when compared with that required to maintain a nonobese state, and that intake must be balanced by energy outgo lest the obesity continue to grow.

Genetics and Early Nutrition in Obesity

The existence of genetic obesity in experimental animals is perhaps the single most startling experimental observation that suggests that more than just human craving for pleasure is involved in the causation of human obesity. A number of rodent strains develops obesity, and one of these, the Zucker obese rat, is startling to behold! The obese animal is enormously large compared with the lean animal. It can, of course, be thinned down by an appropriate diet, but when food is made available ad libitum, the animal eats back to its previous obese state. A predictable number of animals in a given litter will become obese. This prediction is made on purely genetic grounds, and thus the genetic code must be considered the dominant influence in the creation of obesity in this animal. Nevertheless, the obesity cannot come about without an environmental interaction, namely the availability and ingestion of food. Genetic endowment alone, therefore, cannot be the exclusive influence on the level of fat storage.

One also can show that early environmental and nutritional influences will make particularly important and lasting contributions to the level of fat storage in an animal. Thus, newborn rat pups reared in artificially created litters than contain either many siblings or few siblings will receive less or more nutrition, because the mother rat can only produce a limited amount of milk. At weaning, therefore, animals reared in large litters will be smaller than animals reared in small litters; such outcomes are simply the result of competition for food. Such early undernutrition, however, will have lasting effects. The undernourished animal tends to remain perpetually leaner than the initially overfed animal. Do these principles of genetic influence and early nutritional environment pertain to man as well?

Studies of identical and nonidentical twin pairs have been made to evaluate the heritability of human obesity. The startling concordance of obesity in identical twins compared with that in dizygotic or nonidentical twins is strong evidence for a genetic factor operable in human obesity. Although there are, of course, few human experimental data that show the effects of early nutrition as clearly as those that can be obtained with newborn rat pups, some cruel experiments of history have permitted inferences that implicate early nutrition in the later expression of obesity.

In the closing days of World War II, a portion of the southeastern Netherlands was occupied by British and American armies. In the difficult winter of 1944-45, the Netherlands was divided into two portions: that occupied by the Allies and that by the Germans. The nutritional situation was better in the Allied-occupied portion; in fact, the food supply was so scarce in the German-occupied zone that the season was known as the "hunger winter." Approximately 20 years later, the children born during that winter were observed. Cohorts of infants who were either *in utero*, born into the famine, or born after the famine were observed. Infants in the famine zone were compared with those in the area occupied by the Allies. The later incidence of obesity was less in those infants born into the famine compared to those born at the same time in the nonfamine zone, and later obesity was more prevalent in infants who were "protected" from famine by being *in utero* during the famine period. Complex events such as these can be interpreted in many ways, but it is reasonable to assign some role to early nutritional circumstances as a modifier of later body weight in man, similar to that which has been found in experimental animals.

The Energy Equation

Whether on genetic grounds or on the basis of early nutritional experience, the equation $\Delta E = Q - W$ can be solved at different levels of Q and W. In obese people, ΔE may remain at zero for long periods, which indicates that the amount of fat stores is unchanging, even though obesity is present. A ΔE of zero is achieved through an equality between Q and W. When one reduces Q by dietary manipulation, all too often the accompanying reduction in body weight is transient. Reduced-weight obese people tend to regain their lost weight, because an individual in such circumstances will eat to replete adipose stores, so-called eating for "calories" rather than eating for "taste." There is not much evidence that changing the proportion of protein, fat, or carbohydrate or changing the relative sweetness of the diet will alter the re-eating that occurs after weight loss. In fact, the re-eating phenomenon is evidence for the fact that obesity occurs not on the basis of caprice or because of a desire for particularly tasty foods, but rather on behalf of the maintenance of a certain level of body fat storage. Calories from any source are sought to maintain fat storage at a high level in obese people and at another, lower level in lean people.

When an obese individual loses weight under carefully controlled experimental circumstances and is then studied for short periods at a new, lower body weight, it is possible to feed just enough calories to maintain the new lower weight. In this circumstance, ΔE again becomes zero—that is, weight is constant at a normal or near normal level—and Q and W become equal. When Q, the number of calories needed to maintain the new lower body weight, is measured carefully, caloric intake is found to be 15 to 20% below that for never-obese individuals. In other words, after weight reduction in an obese person, there is a persistent state of lowered caloric need, which unfortunately acts to restore the formerly obese state. The lower energy expenditure also has been reported in individuals of normal body weight who have reduced food intake and lost weight to the level of starvation. A conservation of energy outgo opposes any further weight loss.

Several recent studies have suggested that the changes in energy expenditure may occur in those persons who will become obese, even before obesity develops. Studies of members of the Pima tribe living in Arizona, who have a high prevalence of obesity, found low caloric expenditures in people who subsequently became obese. It is as though the first event in the steps that lead to obesity is a reduction in caloric need, which in turn leads to obesity. Obesity occurs first through a reduction in energy outgo, and then through a compensatory hyperphagia, or increase in food intake. If a person who is afflicted with low energy expenditure does not reduce food intake, but rather maintains it at a high level, obesity will surely occur. In some respects, obesity can be considered as "corrective," because the low W, or energy output, rises as the obese state is achieved.

Small numbers of infants born to obese mothers have been studied recently. A few of the infants in such studies will, before showing any undue accumulation of fat, have low thermogenesis, or caloric expenditure. As with the Pimas, this situation is rectified by the assumption of obesity. Energy outgo rises to more normal or expected levels as fat storage rises. A key question for the experimental scientist is how thermogenesis or caloric expenditure and food intake are coupled and, in turn, how these coupled phenomena are related to the total level of fat storage. It would appear that Q and W vary with changes in fat storage, declining at low levels and rising at higher levels of storage. The decline in Q and W is somehow perceived as "starvation" which must be corrected by an increase in Q and the attainment of a new balance of Q and W at a higher level of fat storage.

Fat Cell Metabolism and Other New Factors in Obesity

Fat cells, or adipocytes, have been implicated in these controls. It has been shown that individuals who are markedly obese have a greater number of fat cells; when weight loss occurs, the number of fat cells is unchanged, but the size of the cells is reduced. Is the small fat cell related in any way to the reduction in thermogenesis that occurs in obese persons who have reduced their weight? There is currently no evidence for an affirmative answer to this question, but adipocytes have protein products with various functions. One of these proteins, lipoprotein lipase, assists in the degradation of blood fats and their deposit in adipose tissue; specific functions have not been identified for other, more recently observed proteins such as adipsin. Could such proteins be related to the control of energy metabolism? The evidence is not at hand. The recent ability to culture certain cell lines that transform into adipocytes in vitro gives hope, however, that the nature of fat cell growth and replication will soon be better understood. In such tissue cultures, the products of adipocytes can be measured more directly and observed under controlled experimental circumstances.

Conclusions

There is much more to be learned. The function of the autonomic, or involuntary, nervous system has been implicated in the pathogenesis of obesity. There may be important neuropeptides that alter energy outgo and food intake. Connections among these neuropeptides and with other important regulatory peptides, such as insulin, are objects of careful study at the present time. A better definition of the defect in rodent obesities at the molecular genetic level may provide important clues for unraveling the mystery of the basic biology of obesity.

What is new is the growing evidence that there is a basic biology to obesity. Obesity is not a malevolent or willful behavior without basis in cells, chemicals, or genes. When obesity is understood more fully, we may also have greater insight into whether other behaviors that at present seem willful or even criminal may have a basis in fundamental biology. This may be the most important lesson that obesity can teach us. For now, I only hope that you will believe, as I do, that fat's not fun; it is serious biology.

Suggested Reading

Hirsch J, Leibel RL. New light on obesity [Editorial]. N Engl J Med 1988; 318:509-10.

Hirsch J, Leibel RL. What constitutes a sufficient psychophysiologic explanation for obesity? In: Stunkard AJ, Stellar E, eds. Eating and Its Disorders. New York: Raven Press 1984:124-30.

Leibel RL, Hirsch J. Diminished energy requirements in reduced-obese patients. Metabolism 1984;33:164-70.

2

Adverse Reactions to Food: Facts and Fantasy

RAYMOND SLAVIN, M.D.*

Introduction

The study of food allergies is both topical and controversial. For many years, food allergy was considered a remarkably complex research subject, but recent innovations in investigative techniques have enabled carefully designed studies with which to begin unraveling its complexities. We are now beginning to discover the facts, and these facts should help dispel the myths that have grown up around food allergies.

Food allergy has been known for thousands of years. A famous playwright wrote, "What is one man's poison, señor, is another man's eat or drink," probably one of the first descriptions of food

*St. Louis University School of Medicine, St. Louis, Missouri.

allergy. About 2000 years ago, Ovid, a famous Roman physician, gave what is probably the first advice to allergic patients: "Then there is the matter of food, and I as befits a physician tell you what you should avoid and what you may safely consume."

Controversy Surrounding Food Allergy

The wide range in estimates of the incidence of food allergy demonstrates the controversy that surrounds this subject: the Asthma and Allergy Foundation of America states that less than 1% of the population is allergic to food; the U.S. Department of Agriculture estimates the number at 10 to 15%; and *USA Today* recently stated that 60% of the public has a food allergy.

Several factors account for the existence of such a tremendous disparity: misuse of the word *allergy*, myths about allergy that shape public perception of the illness, careless diagnosis by both physicians and the public, and an unorganized approach to diagnosis. We will briefly examine each of these factors.

Many people call any untoward reaction to food an "allergy." Allergy, however, is only one of several categories of adverse reactions to foods.

Three major myths about allergies continue to be perpetuated. First, many people believe that little scientific knowledge exists about allergies and that we must therefore rely on anecdotal information for diagnosis and treatment. Because of the efforts of many careful investigators throughout the world, however, we are regularly gaining more knowledge about food allergy. The second myth is that no useful test exists for the diagnosis of food allergy. In the diagnosis of true food allergy, however, the skin test is invaluable. The third myth is that food allergy is too complex a subject for meaningful study, but a number of elegant studies recently have revealed much new information.

Careless diagnosis of any adverse reaction to food as a food allergy is a tendency of both the public and physicians. Such carelessness probably accounts for the large statistic quoted by *USA Today* for the number of people who have food allergies.

Many physicians have no organized approach to the diagnosis of food allergy. They often prescribe a diet free from a given food for a few days, then eliminate a different food for a few days, all in a haphazard effort to identify the offending food.

Adverse Food Reactions

Food Intolerance

Food intolerance is a general term for adverse food reactions, which may be divided into four categories: toxic (poisoning), pharmacological, metabolic, and idiosyncratic. Ptomaine poisoning is a toxic food reaction; an adverse reaction occurs to food that has been contaminated by an organism. Some people are extremely sensitive to caffeine, and coffee will keep such a person awake all night as well as cause an extremely rapid heartbeat. Such a response to caffeine is a pharmacological reaction, that is, an exaggerated response to the normal pharmacological effect of a food or food additive. Lactase deficiency (or lactose intolerance) is a metabolic food intolerance; it is particularly prevalent in the black population. Lactase is an intestinal enzyme that breaks down lactose, a sugar present in the milk of mammals. The genetic code of some people does not allow them to produce lactase. If they consume milk or milk products, their inability to break down lactose causes diarrhea and abdominal cramps. An idiosyncratic reaction is a quantitatively abnormal response to a food or an additive that appears to be an allergic reaction, but for which there is no immunological basis. For example, of the 10 million people who have asthma in the United States, 5 to 10% will have an untoward reaction to sulfites, a common additive in wine or on lettuce in fast-food restaurants. No immunological basis exists for the reaction, but sulfites can provoke severe attacks of asthma in some people.

Food Hypersensitivity

Food hypersensitivity, or true food allergy, has a specific immunological basis, and the mechanism by which such a reaction occurs is now well understood. The same mechanism accounts for reactions to ragweed, cats, penicillin, horse serum, and bee venom. The allergic reaction is caused by a (presumably) genetically determined immunoglobulin in blood known as IgE (the allergic antibody). Its production can be stimulated by an inhalant allergen such as ragweed pollen or an ingestant allergen such as cow's milk. IgE attaches to specific cells in the body: mast cells and basophils. When the IgE allergic antibody coats the receptors on a mast cell or basophil, the patient is sensitized, or allergic. The length of a period of sensitization varies widely. The process of sensitization occurs over a period of time through repeated exposure to an allergen. As a consequence of these exposures, the allergic antibody is gradually produced and continues to accumulate. Once a sufficient concentration of antibody has been reached, the IgE attaches to receptors on the basophils and mast cells. On a subsequent exposure to the allergen, a reaction occurs between the antibody on the mast cell and the allergen, which causes the release of substances called mediators from the mast cell or basophil. Mediators, including histamine (which has been known to us the longest) and other substances, have a profound effect on blood vessels, smooth muscle, and mucous glands. The effect of the mediators on shock organs, such as the nose, lungs, skin, or conjunctiva, results in an allergic reaction.

Diagnosis of Food Allergy

Food allergies are easily determined by obtaining a thorough history of the patient, then performing the appropriate diagnostic tests. The most cost-efficient of these is the allergy skin test. The test creates a miniature version of an allergic reaction. Potential allergens—including inhalants (e.g., ragweed pollen, cat dander, house dust), injectants (e.g., penicillin, bee venom), and ingestants (e.g., peanuts, milk protein, wheat)—are suspended in water and placed on the skin in drops. The surface of the skin is broken with a needle, and the allergen penetrates the epidermal barrier and comes into contact with IgE attached to mast cells under the skin. The contact between allergen and antibody releases mediators, most notably histamine, which dilates the nearby blood vessels and increases their permeability. A skin test that is positive for a given allergen will be visible in 15 minutes at the site at which that allergen penetrated the skin. The visible signs of a positive test include swelling and a large area of redness.

In the diagnosis of food allergy, the history of the patient is foremost, but the skin test is very valuable. The skin test has a high negative predictability to food. In other words, a negative skin test is almost absolute evidence that a patient does not have a true food allergy for that allergen. A positive skin test by itself, however, means little. Antibody fixed to the mast cells in the skin in sufficient quantity to produce a positive skin test is not proof that sufficient amounts of IgE antibody exist in the nose, skin, lungs, or gastrointestinal tract to produce a full allergic reaction. A positive skin test, therefore, must always be correlated with the history of the patient.

The best approach for a physician in the diagnosis of food hypersensitivity is to obtain a thorough history in a thoughtful and sympathetic manner. Because food allergy, particularly in adults, is rare, it is also important to maintain a healthy skepticism. A thorough and thoughtful history is necessary to discern hidden sources of foods. It is not enough simply to discover the whole proteins that a patient consumes; the physician must learn everything about the object or substance that caused an allergic reaction.

Let me offer two examples from my own experience. I had a 3-year-old patient who was extremely sensitive to egg. The child had severe systemic reactions; her skin would turn red, and she would wheeze and develop hives. The mother, a nurse, was careful to maintain her daughter on an egg-free diet, and we were sure that would solve the problem. A few weeks later the mother called, absolutely distraught, because her daughter's skin had broken out again in the middle of the afternoon, and the child had had no lunch, only a pretzel. Pretzels seem innocuous enough, but the child's mother did not realize that the substance that makes a pretzel shiny is egg albumen! Another patient, a college student, was highly allergic to peanuts. She avoided them diligently, and one day had a violent reaction after eating chili. She later discovered that peanut paste had been used as a thickener in the chili. These examples represent only a few of the exposures to hidden allergens that a patient may have.

Objective confirmation of the history of an adverse reaction is helpful. When a patient has had a violent, life-threatening reaction to a particular food, it would certainly be unwise to challenge the patient with the food. When the history is inconclusive, however, and objective confirmation is required, the gold standard for diagnosis of food allergy is the double-blinded, placebo-controlled challenge. In such a test, neither the physician nor the patient knows what the patient is receiving, and the patient receives either the food or a placebo in an opaque capsule. Only this type of experiment will absolutely confirm the diagnosis of food allergy.

One must also differentiate hypersensitivity, i.e., allergy, from the other adverse reactions described earlier, namely metabolic, pharmacological, and idiosyncratic. Evidence of specific immunologic sensitization to IgE is best detected by the skin test. The radioimmunoassay, a blood test, measures the amount of IgE directed to a particular food, but a number of good studies have indicated that a radioimmunoassay adds nothing more than great expense to the information obtained from a skin test.

An elimination diet may also be very helpful. In questionable cases, one can put a patient on what allergists call an allergy number 1 diet: lamb, rice, and a few vegetables and fruits. Because so few people in the United States have allergic reactions to lamb, rice, or the fruits and vegetables in this diet, it can be an effective method for diagnosis. If the patient improves, foods are added to the diet, one at a time, every other day, until the allergic symptoms are reproduced. The beauty of such a diet is that only 7 to 10 days are required to determine whether the allergic reaction is a result of a particular food. I emphasize the brevity of that period because some physicians, particularly clinical ecologists, claim that a 6-month period of restricted diet is required to see any results. That claim is absolute nonsense.

A pioneering study was performed at the National Jewish Hospital in Denver, Colorado, by Charles May and Allen Bock, two of the premier investigators in the study of food allergy. The diagnosis of allergy to foods had been made in 81 children. The children were subjected to a double-blinded, placebo-controlled challenge. Only 33% were shown to be positive on such a challenge. May and Bock performed 164 challenge tests and found that only 36 reactions, or 22%, were positive. The positive reactions were in response to peanuts, other nuts, eggs, milk, or soy. Skin tests were positive in the children for every food that caused an allergic reaction. The onset of symptoms ranged between a few minutes and 2 hours, which is important. If a reaction occurs 4 to 8 hours after a meal, it is not likely to be a true food allergy. Finally, the allergic reactions in the children were caused by dried foods in amounts between 20 and 8000 mg. Obviously, an allergic reaction is not an all-or-none phenomenon. Patients often tolerate a food in small amounts but not in larger amounts.

A differential diagnosis is a comparison of the symptoms of two or more similar diseases to determine from which disease the patient is suffering. The differential diagnosis of food allergy would compare its symptoms with those of structural abnormalities, enzyme deficiencies, food contaminants (which could include dyes, preservatives, or toxins), and pharmacological agents (such as tyramine in cheese, alcohol, and caffeine).

Food Allergens

True food allergens, i.e., the foods that cause a majority of the symptoms in true allergic reactions, are few. In children, more than 90% of all food allergies are caused by six substances: eggs, peanuts, milk, fish, soybeans, and wheat. Common allergens in adults include fish, shellfish, tree nuts, peanuts, and eggs. Although chocolate and strawberries are perceived by many people to be allergens, neither food is a common allergen in children or in adults.

The eating habits of a society influence the pattern of food sensitivity. In Sweden, for example, sensitivity to fish is common and sensitivity to nuts is rare, because the Swedes eat a lot of fish but not many nuts. In the United States, rice is a relatively rare cause of food allergy, but in Asian countries, it is a common allergen.

Twenty-five years ago, pediatricians routinely put all milk-sensitive infants on a soy formula, and few of these infants reacted adversely. Over the past 25 years, however, soy has been added to a variety of foods in this country, particularly meats, and allergic reactions to soy have definitely increased. It is now one of the six major food allergens, simply because we eat more of it.

The allergenic fraction, the substance in food that provokes an allergic reaction, is heat-stable and acid-stable and has a high molecular weight. When food is ingested, enzymes, including amylase, pepsin, pancreatic enzymes, and intestinal peptidases, break the food down into smaller metabolic products. In general, the smaller the molecular weight of a substance, the less likely it is to cause an allergic reaction. Patients who lack certain enzymes or whose gastrointestinal tract is more permeable, such as young children, are unable to break down certain food substances and therefore have a greater incidence of allergic diseases. The fact that the gastrointestinal tract in young children is not fully developed is thought to be the reason that so many children develop allergies. As the gastrointestinal tract matures, digestion becomes more complete, and the body is presented with substances of smaller molecular weight.The chances for developing an allergy then become markedly decreased.

Allergic Symptoms

Psychological Influences

A classic study from the early 1950s demonstrates the power that our minds can have over the physical manifestations of an illness. The investigator studied a young woman who believed that she was sensitive to milk. The physician had some doubt and therefore devised a careful study. Her symptoms included pain, abdominal spasm, rapid heart rate, and changes in blood pressure. He inserted a nasogastric tube and told her that she was receiving a placebo, but in fact fed her milk. He then told her she was receiving milk, but gave her instead the placebo. When he gave her the placebo, but told her it was milk, she had abdominal contractions that were absolutely verified, a rapid heart rate, and a drop in blood pressure. When she thought she was receiving the placebo but was in fact receiving milk, she had none of the symptoms. She perceived her sensitivity so definitely that she controlled her autonomic nervous system to cause the documented physiological reactions to appear. This demonstrates how powerful our minds are.

Substantiated Symptoms

Double-blinded, placebo-controlled challenges have substantiated a number of symptoms in food allergy, including generalized anaphylaxis, a severe, life-threatening reaction. If a patient's history suggests anaphylaxis, the patient is not ordinarily challenged. Some intrepid investigators have done so, however, and have caused generalized anaphylaxis with cardiovascular collapse and in some cases cardiorespiratory arrest. Also, anaphylaxis sometimes is associated with exercise. Well-documented cases exist in which a particular food was ingested, after which the person exercised vigorously and suffered a severe systemic reaction. In such cases, if the patient ate the food but did not exercise, there was no reaction; likewise, exercise with no ingestion of the food did not produce a reaction. The first such report involved celery, usually a nonallergenic food; the second involved shellfish, which is highly allergenic.

Other symptoms that have been substantiated by blinded challenge are skin manifestations (e.g., hives), nasal and bronchial respiratory symptoms. A recent study of patients with migraine headaches suggested that food may be the cause in 20 to 30% of these patients. Gastrointestinal symptoms that have been substantiated by blinded challenges include immediate reactions such as nausea, abdominal pain, cramps, vomiting, and diarrhea. Manifestations may also be simply an itching of the mouth or swelling of the tongue.

Unsubstantiated Symptoms

Symptoms that never have been substantiated by blinded challenges include central nervous system reactions, learning disorders, and hyperactivity. In the famous "Twinkie case," a murderer claimed that he was addicted to Twinkies and that the sugar in the product altered his behavior. None of the aforementioned conditions has ever been shown to be the result of a food allergy. In a recent study, a large group of children who had been diagnosed hyperactive as a result of sugar were subjected to a double-blinded, placebo-controlled study. The children showed no more hyperactivity with sugar than with the placebo. Other conditions that have never been substantiated include the tension-fatigue syndrome and arthritis.

Food Additives

Many food additives have been cited as possible causes of food allergy. Some of these include preservatives (e.g., benzoate), stabilizers, conditioners, thickening agents (e.g., gums), sweetening agents, food coloring, flavoring agents, antioxidants (e.g., sulfites), and many miscellaneous additives.

Additives that commonly have been claimed to be associated with adverse reactions include: FD & C dyes (particularly yellow #5), various parabens (commonly used as preservatives), BHA and BHT, nitrates, nitrites, monosodium glutamate, various sulfites, sulfur dioxide, sodium and potassium sulfite, bisulfite and metabisulfite, and aspartame.

Tartrazine yellow dye was incriminated some time age as a supposedly common cause of hives. The reaction was believed to be particularly common in patients who were allergic to aspirin. Aspirin is the second most common drug responsible for untoward reactions. (Penicillin is first.) A reaction to aspirin is a bona fide drug reaction, not an allergic or true allergic reaction based on IgE, but it can be devastating nonetheless. It was previously thought that 10 to 15% of all people who were allergic to aspirin were also allergic to tartrazine. The early reports were largely anecdotal, and their poorly controlled study designs were a result of both a lack of double-blinded placebo control and a choice of inappropriate criteria for a positive reaction. More recent studies have indicated that the prevalence of reactivity is very rare.

Adverse reactions to sulfites led to regulation of their use; as of 1985, any product that contained more than 10 parts per million had to be labeled so that sulfite-sensitive people can determine from a label whether sulfites are present. Sulfites are not allowed in red meats. Sulfites had been used in restaurants to keep lettuce, avocados, and potatoes from turning brown. That use was banned in August 1986, and in January 1988, all wines that contained sulfites had to be so labeled. Some sources of sulfites include salad bars, dried fruit, processed package foods, shrimp, and wine. Sensitivity to sulfur dioxide, a by-product of sulfite degradation, has been suggested as a mechanism to explain reactions to sulfite. A few people seem to lack an enzyme, sulfite-oxidase, that breaks down sulfites to inactivate sulfates. A true allergic, IgE-mediated reaction is rare, but might be the cause of non-asthmatic response to sulfites, such as hives, swelling, or anaphylactic reaction.

Reactions to parabens and benzoates, common preservatives and antioxidants, have been reported. The majority of the reported reactions, however, are not well documented.

There have been claims of reactions to other additives, including aspartame, various antioxidants, nitrates, and nitrites. A reaction to aspartame, reported in the *Annals of Internal Medicine,* involved a subject who was studied with pure aspartame. More recently, Metcalfe and his group from the National Institutes of Health reported that they were not able to reproduce alleged aspartame-related allergic reactions in 12 individuals after blinded challenges with aspartame. There are unsubstantiated claims that monosodium glutamate, a flavor enhancer used in Chinese restaurants, is associated with the Chinese restaurant syndrome, which consists of flushing, headaches, and abdominal pain.

Appropriate Procedures for the Scientific Investigation of Food Allergy

Clinical trials and double-blinded, placebo-controlled challenges are the real basis for a medically reasoned judgment. Specific steps should be followed to establish the validity of any procedure, whether diagnostic or therapeutic. One should start with a clearly defined and reproducible hypothesis. Procedures and materials should be reported so that other investigators can repeat the study. The characteristics of the subject should be described. Subjects must be randomly assigned, in a double-blind fashion, to test and control groups of the appropriate size. Data must be evaluated objectively, analyzed by the appropriate statistical methods, and the study should be prepared for peer review and publication.

Unfortunately, our colleagues in clinical ecology do not follow this procedure. Rather than present their views for scientific scrutiny, they go directly to the lay press, where they claim that food sensitivity can account for a myriad of problems, including compulsive alcohol consumption, hyperactivity, asthma, hypertension, and schizophrenia.

Conclusion

Why are so many people convinced that they have a food allergy? First, I think that orthodox medical management too often fails people who complain of a food allergy. Conventional physicians are often disorganized in their approach to food allergy, and physicians sometimes refer these people elsewhere without taking the time to examine a problem thoroughly. Second, misleading information is too readily available. One can hardly pick up a magazine or newpaper, even a reliable newspaper, without reading that food allergy is at the root of most of man's ills. Third, people prefer a physical diagnosis to a psychological diagnosis. Several studies have shown that patients who respond to an evangelistic, total-elimination-diet approach have a high incidence of psychoneurosis. It is, of course, always easier to blame our problems on an outside influence rather than something intrinsic. Finally, food has many emotional connotations, which may cause people to believe that they are allergic.

Very good investigators, who are designing excellent studies, are now devoting themselves to the subject of food allergy. I have no doubt that over the next few years, as this subject is further unraveled, we will see even more facts and much less fantasy.

Suggested Reading

Anderson JA. The establishment of common language concerning adverse reactions to foods and food additives. J Allergy Clin Immunol 1986;78:140.

Bock SA. A critical evaluation of clinical trials in adverse reactions to foods in children. J Allergy Clin Immunol 1986;78:165.

Kettelhut BV, Metcalfe DD. Adverse reactions to foods. In: Middleton E Jr et al, eds. Allergy: Principles and Practice, 3rd ed. St. Louis: CV Mosby, 1988:Chapter 63.

3

Fats and Food Acceptance

ADAM DREWNOWSKI, Ph.D.*

Introduction

The diet of Western societies is regarded as overly high in refined sugars and fat. According to nutritional surveys, fats account for up to 38% of daily calories in the typical American diet, while sugars contribute a further 12%. The average adult consumes between 64 and 98 grams of fat (Figure 1) and an estimated 53 grams of added sugars per day.

Among the chief sources of dietary fat are meat, fats and cooking oils, and dairy products, including milk, cheese, and frozen desserts. Added sugars, mainly sucrose and fructose, are provided by discretionary table use, sweetened beverages, bakery goods, and confectionery products. Sweet desserts whose chief ingredients are

*University of Michigan School of Public Health, Ann Arbor, Michigan.

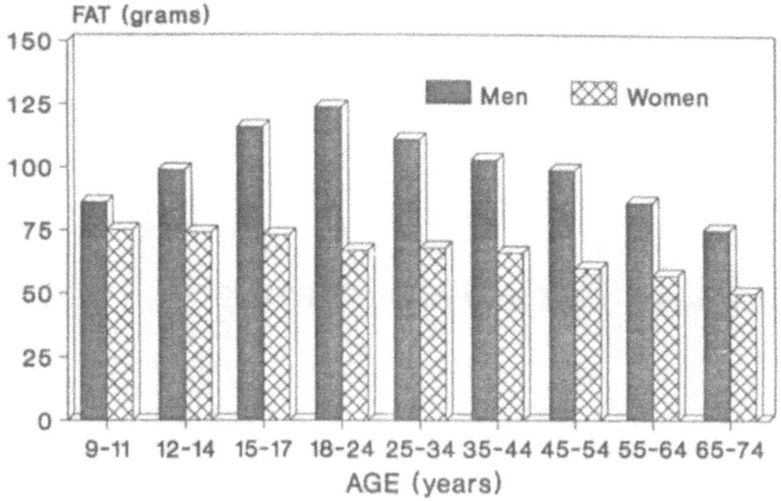

Figure 1 Nutrient composition of the average American adult's diet. Fat intake in grams per day for persons aged 9 to 74 years. (U.S. NHANES II data, 1976-1980.)

sugar and fat seem to fall in a special category. Commonly thought of as sweet, carbohydrate-rich foods, cookies, ice cream, and chocolate often derive the bulk of their calories from fat. The fat and sugar content of chocolate products typically accounts for 80 to 98% of total calories. Other products containing both sugar and fat include cakes, cookies, pies, milk-based beverages, and a range of frozen desserts.

Sweet, fat-rich desserts are not only uniquely palatable, but also may be uniquely fattening. As several studies with laboratory rats have shown, prolonged feeding of diets rich in sugar or fat leads to hyperphagia and diet-induced obesity in susceptible rat strains. Diets containing both sugar and fat appear to be most effective in promoting weight gain. A combination of sweetened condensed milk and chocolate chip cookies promotes obesity more effectively than do 32% sucrose solutions or vegetable oil mixed with standard laboratory chow. Recent data from Japan further indicate that ingestion of sugar/fat mixtures promotes greater deposition of body fat in rats than do equicaloric amounts of sugar and fat consumed separately at different times of day.

What mechanisms are responsible for the development and maintenance of human preferences for sweet, high-fat foods? Preliminary evidence suggests that a combination of metabolic, sensory, and attitudinal factors may be involved.

Food Preferences and Food Cravings

Scientific literature on the nature of food preferences has been dominated by reports of cravings for carbohydrate-rich foods. Such cravings, said to be provoked by an imbalance of a central neurotransmitter, serotonin, have been reported among obese patients, bulimic women, and depressed individuals suffering from seasonal affective disorder. Because carbohydrate ingestion (in the absence of protein) stimulates serotonin synthesis in the rat brain, the consumption of carbohydrate snacks by humans has been reported to increase satiety, relieve depression, and promote a sense of well-being.

The key assumption of the serotonin hypothesis has been that cravings are directed at a specific macronutrient—carbohydrate—and not at any particular food item. Sensory aspects of carbohydrate snacks likewise were dismissed as unimportant. It should be noted, however, that the typical objects of "carbohydrate craving" are chocolate, ice cream, cookies, pastries, and other desserts, all foods in which the chief source of carbohydrate is simple sugar, usually presented in combination with dietary fat. In some laboratory studies, carbohydrate cravers were identified on the basis of their liking for chocolate bars, chocolate cupcakes, and candies. In other studies, cakes, frozen pastries, and even an ice cream sundae topped with whipped cream were classified as carbohydrate-rich foods. As simple nutritional analysis reveals, these foods contain sugar, but are also rich in dietary fat.

Why is fat the forgotten ingredient of sweet, high-fat foods? As shown in Figure 2, fat is an important component of ice cream and chocolate. However, studies on food acceptance generally have equated palatability with sweet taste. It should be recognized that the fat content of food also plays an important sensory role. For example, such desirable attributes of ice cream as its richness, smoothness, and creaminess are linked directly to the presence of butter

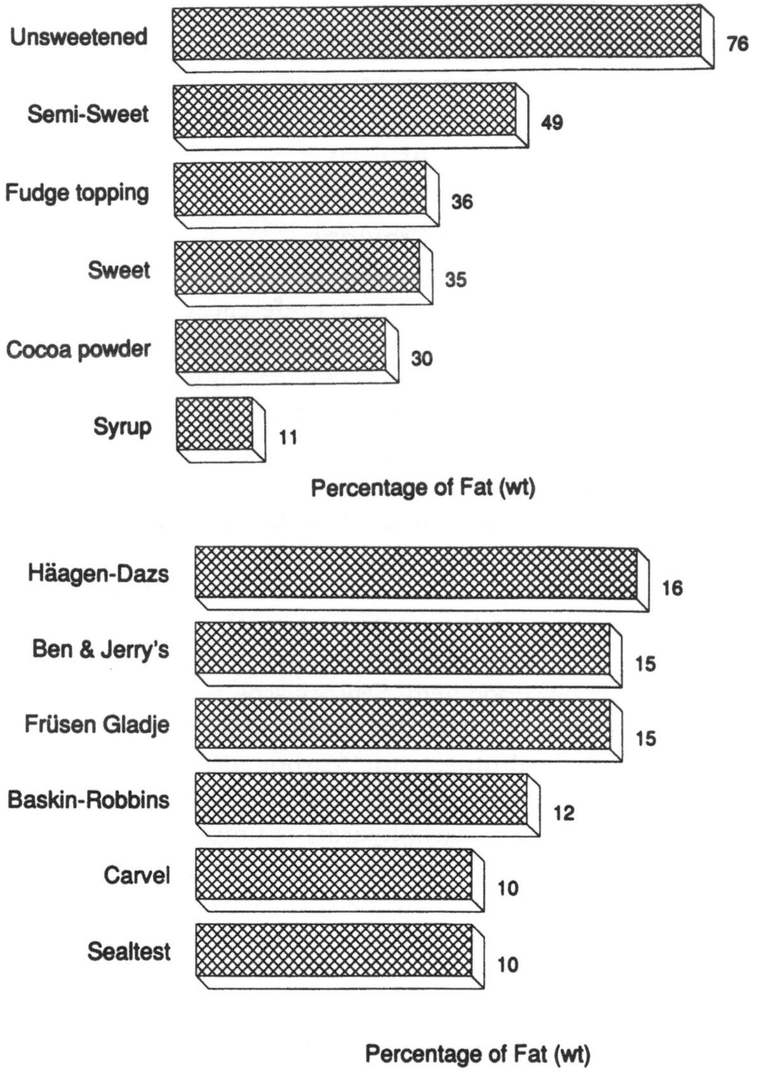

Figure 2 Fat content (percentage wt/wt) of (top) chocolate and (bottom) ice cream. (Data for Hershey Products from Hershey Foods Corp.)

fat. Fat endows ice cream with its characteristic mouthfeel and prevents the formation of ice crystals. Premium ice cream contains between 16 and 18% butterfat, as opposed to 10-12% for standard-grade products. Many consumers who like the premium product, however, are unaware of its elevated fat content. Similarly, the fat content of chocolate is not necessarily obvious to the consumer; since no single sensory attribute can be associated unambiguously with product fatness, attention is often focused on the other chief ingredient.

Sensory Evaluation Studies

Laboratory studies on taste responsiveness have generally focused on the perception of sweetness and the development of preferences for sweet taste. Relatively few studies have explored sensory perception of fats in sweetened foods, or the role fats play in determining food acceptance.

Sensory evaluation studies have shown that hedonic preferences for sweet solutions or sweet foods generally follow an inverted-U curve. The hedonic optimum or breakpoint is in the range of 8 to 10% sucrose in water, and is somewhat higher for solid foods. We also know that individual hedonic profiles are highly variable: Some subjects prefer, while other dislike, sugar solutions of increasing intensity of sweetness. At one time, sweetness preferences were thought to be an accurate index of the energy repletion of the organism. Attempts to link taste preferences to body weight status, however, have been largely unsuccessful. Studies using sucrose solutions, sweetened beverages, and chocolate milkshakes found no consistent relationship between sweet taste preferences and overweight. Large-scale consumer studies found no relationship between body weight and hedonic preferences for increasing concentrations of sugar in such foods as apricot nectar, canned peaches, lemonade, or vanilla ice cream.

Perception of Fat in Foods

The study of fat in food is considerably more complicated than the study of sugar solutions. Fats provide the characteristic texture, flavor, and aroma of many foods and endow foods with a variety of textural characteristics. Oral perception of fats seems to be mediated primarily through texture and mouthfeel, and to a lesser degree through olfaction. Because fats are associated with a wide range of product textures, however, it is not always clear what oral sensations contribute to the perception of fat content.

As a result, sensory assessment of fat in foods relies on a wide range of attribute scales. Which of the many possible attributes is most closely linked to stimulus fat content? The answer seems to depend on the nature of the food system. Past sensory evaluation studies of such foods as peanut butter, margarine, and mayonnaise have established that mouthfeel attributes of thickness, smoothness, and creaminess are all linked to the perception of fat content. In liquid dairy products where fat is contained in emulsified globules, the perception of fatness is largely guided by stimulus smoothness, thickness, or viscosity. Elsewhere, the mouthfeel of beverages has been described in such terms as thick, creamy, heavy, syrupy, and viscous. The fat content of foods has also been linked to such terms as hard, soft, juicy, chewy, greasy, viscous, slippery, creamy, crisp, crunchy, and brittle. It should be noted that many attributes in the terminology of food texture are not hedonically neutral. Although creaminess may be a desirable property in many foods, greasiness and sliminess generally are not.

Systematic evaluation of food texture began with a classic body of work, the General Foods Texture Profile. Texture evaluation was viewed as a dynamic analysis of the mechanical, geometrical, fat, and moisture aspects of foods, occurring along the dimension of time, from first bite through complete mastication. The primary mechanical characteristics of food were defined as hardness, cohesiveness, adhesiveness, and viscosity, while secondary characteristics were brittleness, chewiness, and gumminess. Geometrical characteristics were defined as those related to the shape, size, and orientation of food particles (e.g., gritty, grainy, coarse), while mouthfeel characteristics were related to the perception of moisture or fat.

The Texture Profile introduced a number of anchored rating scales, each referenced to an array of physical standards. For example, the standard viscosity scale (shown in Table 1) represented eight degrees of viscosity, each defined by a commercially available product. As can be seen, over half the standards are foods containing

Table 1 The Standard Viscosity Scale

Rating	Product	Brand or manufacturer	Sample (tsp)
1	Water	Crystal Spring	1/2
2	Light cream	Sealtest Foods	1/2
3	Heavy cream	Sealtest Foods	1/2
4	Evaporated milk	Carnation Co.	1/2
5	Maple syrup	F. H. Leggett & Co.	1/2
6	Chocolate syrup	Hershey Foods Corp.	1/2
7	Mixture: 1/2 cup mayonnaise and 2 tbs heavy cream	Best Foods—Hellman's and Sealtest Foods	1/2
8	Condensed milk	Borden Foods Magnolia Brand	1/2

Source: Adapted from Szczesniak et al., 1963.

different amounts of fat. Similarly, the adhesiveness scale included such standards as Crisco oil, cream cheese, and peanut butter.

Although the assessment of fat content in liquids is probably guided by stimulus viscosity, different textural cues may be associated with the presence of fat in solids. In some cases, fatlike stimulus texture can be achieved in the absence of actual fat. In a recent study, 50 young women rated the sweetness and fat content of 15 stimuli resembling cake frostings. The samples were composed of sucrose (range 20 to 77% wt/wt), polydextrose (a bland, partly metabolizable starch), unsalted butter (range 15 to 35% wt/wt), and distilled water. As expected, the perception of sweetness intensity was a function only of sucrose levels. In contrast, the oral assessment of fat content was largely mediated by product texture. Fatness ratings were a combined function of three ingredients: fat, polydextrose, and water. The addition of sugar caused a sharp decrease in fatness ratings and the sweetest stimuli were perceived as lowest in fat. This observation may help explain why fat is often the invisible component of sweet, high-fat desserts, with most of the attention being focused on the sweet taste of sugar.

The relationship between food texture and the perception of fat content has major implications for the use of fat substitutes in reduced-calorie food products. The reliance on texture cues in sensory assessment of fats means that an illusion of fat content can be created by making the stimulus more viscous, by either gelling or using of hydrocolloid thickeners. A newly developed fat substitute, Simplesse®, consists of microparticulated protein designed to emulate the mouthfeel of cream or fat.

Preferences for Fat in Food

The relationship between perceived fat content and food acceptance is fairly complex. The fat content of liquid dairy products often serves as an index of product quality and thus is linked to food acceptance. However, consumers may also express preferences for high-fat foods, especially solids, without being aware of the elevated fat content. Acceptability ratings may also be influenced by habitual patterns of use and by cognitive attitudes toward fats, given that fat-rich foods are generally perceived as unhealthy.

Our early studies calibrated relative sensory preferences for sugar versus fat. A series of clinical studies with mixtures of milk, cream, and sugar tested the hypothesis that taste responsiveness is a biological marker that may help discriminate between populations at extremes of body weight. The studies were conducted with anorectic and bulimic patients and with massively obese women enrolled in a program for weight reduction. Additional responses were obtained from groups of age-matched normal-weight female controls. Subject characteristics are summarized in Table 2.

Table 2 Subject Characteristics and Hedonic Optima for Sucrose and Fat

Subject group	*n*	Age (yr)	Weight (kg)	Sucrose (%)	Fat (%)
Obese	12	38.0	95.8	4.4	34.5
Reduced obese	8	32.7	67.9	10.1	35.1
Normal-weight	15	30.1	58.8	7.7	20.7
Normal-weight	16	19.1	57.7	9.1	28.7
Bulimic	7	19.4	56.8	15.3	27.9
Anorectic	25	17.2	40.5	12.7	16.5

Source: Adapted from Drewnowski et al., 1985, 1987.

The subjects rated the sweetness, creaminess, and fat content of chilled sugar/fat mixtures and judged the acceptability of each sample on a nine-point category scale. The use of a mathemetical modeling technique known as the Response Surface Method (RSM) helped to predict the shape of hedonic or pleasure response for a wide range of stimulus ingredient levels. Hedonic response surface obtained for a group of normal-weight adults is shown in Figure 3. The data are presented as a three-dimensional projection (left panel) and as corresponding or isohedonic contours (right panel).

Hedonic response profiles were strongly interactive. Although the acceptability of sweetened skim milk or unsweetened milk or cream was relatively low, the combination of cream and sugar produced a powerful hedonic synergy. The RSM model predicted highest preference ratings for a mixture containing 20% fat and 8% sugar. As shown in Table 2, the optimal sugar and fat levels varied among subject groups. Obese women tended to prefer stimuli that were rich in fat but relatively low in sugar. In contrast, anorectic women liked sweetness but tended to avoid those stimuli that were rich in fat.

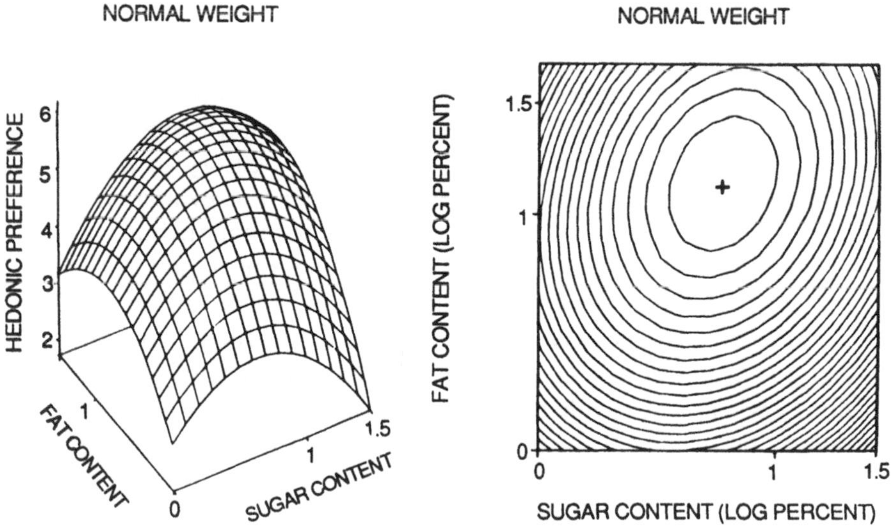

Figure 3 Acceptability of sugar/fat mixtures. Hedonic response surface expressed as a three-dimensional projection (left) or as iso-preference contours (right). Region of optimal preference is denoted by +.

The dislike for fat among dieters may be influenced by metabolic factors, or may be modulated by previous experience contingent on a number of attitudinal, social, or cultural variables.

Regulatory Mechanisms

Preferences and cravings for sweet carbohydrates are thought to be triggered by physiological or metabolic events. One possibility, prominently mentioned in the literature, is serotonin imbalance. However, the typical targets of carbohydrate craving are not bland starches, vegetables, or bread, but palatable sweet desserts that are generally composed of sugar and fat. Clearly, the sensory aspects of such foods are an essential part of their appeal.

The serotonin hypothesis ignores the hedonic aspects of appetite. A different approach that is more sensitive to sensory factors and the pleasure response to foods involves endogenous opioid peptides, pleasure-enhancing molecules manufactured by the human brain. In several studies with rats and mice, intakes of sugar and fat have been linked to the endogenous opioid peptide system. Dietary studies have further shown that morphine-injected animals selectively increase fat intake, while the opioid antagonist naltrexone blocks overeating induced by a palatable cafeteria diet. Preliminary data further indicate that the opioid system may influence pleasure response to the taste of sugar and fat mixtures. Sensory acceptability of chilled mixtures of milk, cream, and sugar was evaluated after intravenous infusions of opioid agonist butorphanol, but was reduced by naloxone. Naloxone also reduced the consumption of chocolate and cookies, resulting in a significantly reduced fat intake.

Preferences for sweet, high-fat foods are learned through associations between taste and the positive consequences of food ingestion. Foods that provide a rapid influx of calories may be especially rewarding to the organism. Some investigators have made the distinction between innate preferences for the sweet taste of sugar, which are present at birth, and preferences for high-fat foods, which might be learned during childhood or adolescence. For example, the diet of infants and children is typically rich in sugar and fat.

Children love sweets, and the consumption of sugar per kilogram body weight is far greater in childhood than it is during adolescence or in adult life. It might be argued that sugar is the chief vehicle for the introduction of fat into the child's diet. Fat is a component of milk-based formulas, sweet desserts, and even peanut butter and jelly. As preferences for sweet taste and sugar consumption decline between childhood and adolescence, fat continues to provide between 36 and 40% of daily calories throughout the life cycle.

Attitudinal Factors

Food acceptance is also influenced by social norms. A survey of food preferences conducted with the U.S. Armed Forces showed milk, grilled steak, and French fries to be the most highly preferred foods. These foods are typical of the American diet, and all are relatively rich in fat. In contrast, foods that were associated with dieting (e.g., skim milk, diet soda, and fruit yogurt) tended to be rated as unacceptable by Army personnel.

Not everyone, however, accepts a high-fat diet. Some individuals, especially women dieters, select low-fat foods. Although high-fat foods may be more appealing, food acceptance is influenced not only by sensory factors, but also by a wide range of psychological and attitudinal variables. Most dramatic examples of interaction between taste factors, attitudes, and behavior are found among women with eating disorders—anorexia nervosa and bulimia.

In sensory evaluation studies, anorectic patients liked intensely sweet stimuli but disliked foods rich in fat. According to some clinical reports, anorectic women were willing to eat vegetables, lettuce, fresh fruit, cheese, and sometimes eggs, but were disgusted by milk and meat. Although the pattern of food selection in eating disorders has been described as a "carbohydrate phobia," fat avoidance seems closer to the mark. Sweet, high-fat foods, such as chocolate and ice cream, appear to be consumed only in the course of uncontrollable eating binges that are invariably followed by self-induced vomiting.

Fat avoidance may have a physiological or a psychological basis. One possibility is prior conditioning and the pairing of fat odors with bouts of nausea or vomiting. Fat-protein mixtures, in particular, are avoided by pregnant women and by patients undergoing chemotherapy. Another possibility is that eating-disorder patients primarily avoid foods high in calories, that is, foods rich in fat. Anorectic patients show a rigid attitude, allowing themselves to eat only those foods that they also perceive as nutritious and low in calories. Fat-containing foods are regarded as forbidden, and anorectic patients often rate vegetables as preferable to ice cream.

Conclusions

The consumption of dietary fats in the form of sweet, high-fat desserts is influenced by a range of factors, including metabolic, sensory, and attitudinal variables. Taste seems to be a central factor in mediating food acceptance, and sugar/fat mixtures exert a powerful hedonic appeal. Preliminary evidence suggests that endogenous opiates might be involved in mediating the pleasure response to sweet, high-fat foods. However, physiological factors do not wholly explain the connection between fats and food acceptance. Although fats provide the variety, richness, and texture in the diet, attitudes toward high-fat foods are not always uniformly positive. Many consumers view fats as the chief source of unwanted calories and deliberately avoid high-fat foods.

Fats have been identified as the chief problem nutrient in the American diet. Dietary recommendations routinely include the advice to reduce daily fat intake from the present average of 38% to a more acceptable level of 25 to 30% of daily calories. How is such reduction to be accomplished? The Surgeon General's 1988 report suggests the selection of lean meats, fish, and low-fat diary products, and increased consumption of vegetables and fruit. However, low-fat diets tend to be bland, and adherence to low-fat diets is a common problem in the dietary management of hyperlipidemias. The main challenge for nutritionists and the food industry is to reduce fat calories while preserving the sensory appeal and the palatability of the diet.

Suggested Reading

Blass EM. Opioids, sugar and the inherent taste of sweet: broad motivational implications. In: Dobbing J, ed. Sweetness. Berlin: Springer-Verlag, 1987:115-24.

Block G, Dresser CM, Hartman AM, Carroll MD. Nutrient sources in the American diet: quantitative data from the NHANES II survey. Am J Epidemiol 1985;122:27-40.

Brandt MA, Skinner EZ, Coleman JA. Texture profile method. J Food Sci 1963;28:404-9.

Cooper HR. Texture in dairy products and its sensory evaluation. In: Moskowitz HR, ed. Food Texture. New York: Marcel Dekker, 1987: 251-72.

Cussler EL, Kokini JL, Weinheimer RL, Moskowitz HR. Food texture in the mouth. Food Technol 1979;33:89-92.

Drewnowski A. Sweetness and obesity. In: Dobbing J, ed. Sweetness. Berlin: Springer-Verlag, 1987.

Drewnowski A. Fats and food texture: sensory and hedonic evaluations. In: Moskowitz HR, ed. Food Texture. New York: Marcel Dekker, 1987:217-50.

Drewnowski A. Sensory preferences for fat and sugar in adolescence and adult life. In: Murphy C, Cain WS, Hegsted DM, eds. Ann NY Acad Sci 1989;561:243-9.

Drewnowski A, Greenwood MRC. Cream and sugar: human preferences for high-fat foods. Physiol Behav 1983;30:629-33.

Drewnowski A, Brunzell JD, Sande K, Iverius Ph, Greenwood MRC. Sweet tooth reconsidered: taste preferences in human obesity. Physiol Behav 1985;35:617-22.

Drewnowski A, Halmi KA, Pierce B, Gibbs J, Smith GP. Taste and eating disorders. Am J Clin Nutr 1987;46:422-50.

Drewnowski A, Shrager EE, Lipsky C, Stellar E, Greenwood MRC. Sugar and fat: sensory and hedonic evaluations of liquid and solid foods. Physiol Behav 1989;45:177-83.

Drewnowski A, Schwartz M. Invisible fats: sensory assessment of sugar/fat mixtures. Appetite 1990;14:203-17.

Glinsman WH, Irausquin H, Park YK. Evaluation of health aspects of sugars contained in carbohydrate sweeteners. J Nutr 1986;116:S1-216.

Jowitt R. The terminology of food texture. J Text Stud 1974;5:351-8.

Kokini JL, Kadane JB, Cussler EL. Liquid texture perceived in the mouth. J Text Stud 1977;8:195-218.

Lieberman HR, Wurtman JJ, Chew B. Changes in mood after carbohydrate consumption among obese individuals. Am J Clin Nutr 1986; 44:772-8.

Meiselman HL, Waterman D, Symington LE. Armed Forces Food Preferences. Tech Rep 75-63-FSL. Natick, MA: US Army Natick Development Center, 1974.

Mela DJ. Sensory assessment of fat content in fluid dairy products. Appetite 1988;10:37-44.

Midkiff EE, Bernstein IL. Targets of learned food aversions in humans. Physiol Behav 1985;34:839-41.

Moskowitz HR, Kluter RA, Westerling J, Jacobs HL. Sugar sweetness and pleasantness: evidence for different psychophysical laws. Science 1974; 184:583-5.

Pangborn RM, Bos KE, Stern J. Dietary fat intake and taste responses to fat in milk by under-, normal-, and overweight women. Appetite 1985;6:25-40.

Pangborn RM, Dunkley WL. Sensory discrimination of fat and solids-not-fat in milk. J Dairy Sci 1964;47:719-25.

Paykel ES, Mueller PS, de la Vergne PM. Amitryptyline, weight gain and carbohydrate craving: a side effect. Br J Psychiatr 1973;125: 501-7.

Rosenthal NE, Genhart M, Jacobsen FM, Skwerer RG, Wehr TA. Disturbance of appetite and weight regulation in seasonal affective disorder. Ann NY Acad Sci 1987;499:216-30.

Schneeman BO. Fats in the diet: why and where? Food Technol 1986; 10:115-20.

Shepherd R, Stockley L. Fat consumption and attitudes toward food with a high fat content. Hum Nutr: Appl Nutr 1985;39A:431-42.

The Surgeon General's Report on Nutrition and Health. DHHS (PHS) Publ No 88-50210. Washington, DC: US Government Printing Office, 1988.

Suzuki M, Tamura T. Intake timing of fat and insulinogenic sugars and efficiency of body fat accumulation. In: Bray GA et al, eds. Diet and obesity. Tokyo: Japan Scientific Soc Press, 1988.

Szczesniak AS, Brandt MA, Friedman HH. Development of standard rating scales for mechanical parameters of texture and correlations between the objective and the sensory methods of texture evaluation. J Food Sci 1963;28:497-503.

Szczesniak AS. Consumer awareness of texture and other food attributes. II. J Text Stud 1971;2:196-206.

Thompson DA, Moskowitz HR, Campbell R. Effects of body weight and food intake on pleasantness ratings for a sweet stimulus. J Appl Psychol 1976;41:77-83.

Tuorila H, Pangborn RM. Prediction of reported consumption of selected fat-containing foods. Appetite 1988;11:81-95.

Weiffenbach JM, Ed. Taste and Development: The Genesis of Sweet Preference. DHEW Publ No (NIH) 77-1068. Bethesda, MD: US Government Printing Office, 1977.

Wurtman JJ, Wurtman RJ, Growdon JH, Henry P, Lipscomb A, Zeisel SH. Carbohydrate craving in obese people: suppression by treatments affecting serotoninergic transmission. Int J Eating Dis 1981;1:2-15.

4

Nutrition and Aging

IRWIN ROSENBERG, M.D.*

Introduction

By the year 2000, one person in five in the United States will be over the age of 65. This is a striking change from the demographics at the turn of the century, when one person in 25 was over the age of 65. Life expectancy then was 47 years compared with 74 years today. These changes are similar to those in other industrial nations, and similar changes are beginning to occur in the developing countries. The greater life expectancy is certainly representative of our ability as a society to make advances in technology, health care, and delivery of nutrition. However, the massive demographic shift just described, from a population that is mostly young to one that includes a large number of old and very old people, presents humankind with one of its most dramatic challenges.

*USDA Human Nutrition Center on Aging, Tufts University, Boston, Massachusetts.

Not only are there striking differences between people in their 70s compared with those in their 90s, but 70-year-olds are far more different from one another than is true at younger ages in the life cycle. Chronological and biological age in the same person may be very different. Although there will be an increase in the number of persons over 70 and even over 80 who are vigorous, vital, and independent, there likewise will be more persons who are chronically ill, dependent, and institutionalized. Chronic conditions, as well as dementia, prevent functional independence and increase the need for dietary services and other kinds of long-term care. For example, in 1985 more than 5 million persons over age 65 needed special care to remain independent, and this number is expected to exceed 7 million by the year 2000. It has been estimated that nearly 3 million older Americans who do not live in institutions still require assistance with the basic activities of food consumption, including shopping, meal preparation, and eating. One survey has estimated that 75% of all patients who receive home health care require therapeutic diets and could benefit from the services of trained nutrition professionals.

Our challenge is to work toward a society and environment that enable the greatest number of our elders to lead vigorous, fulfilling, and independent lives. Nutrition must play an important part in meeting that challenge, just as advances in the quality and availability of food have contributed to longer life expectancy.

Nutrition for Older People: Issues That Require Study

How can nutrition play a part in increasing the well-being of our older population? First we must understand better the processes behind the age-related decline in the efficiency of many of our critical functions that begins in middle age. No decline is more functionally significant than the decline in lean body mass, which is associated with a reciprocal increase in body fat. The decline in bone mass with age has received a tremendous amount of attention, particularly with regard to osteoporosis and its effects on the elderly. Consider, however, the implication of the decrease in muscle mass with respect to the behavior of the elderly. Have we given it enough attention? Perhaps it needs a name. I suggest, from Greek, *sarcomalacia* ("softening of the flesh") or *sarcopenia* ("lack of flesh"). If we identified this decline by name, we might study it more thoroughly, particularly its relationship to exercise, which we have now begun to do. We know that elders can build and rebuild muscle mass. Even the frail elderly can improve function by a remarkable 180% on a short exercise regimen. No single feature of age-related decline can more dramatically affect calorie intake, overall nutrient intake and status, breathing, ambulation, mobility, and independence than the decline in muscle mass. Increased attention to this process would pay off in the increased health and vigor of older people.

At the USDA Human Nutrition Research Center at Tufts University, our mission is to understand the basis for the age-related decline in the efficiency of critical human functions. From this understanding we devise dietary and nutritional strategies that, along with other interventions such as exercise, can be instituted earlier in life. Such interventions will reduce the rate and severity of this decline and result in more vigorous, fulfilled, and independent older people. These people will then be less dependent on chronic medical care and institutionalization. The other challenge in our mission is to understand how the inevitable changes in physiology influence the requirement for nutrients so that at any age a diet based on such understanding, properly defined and administered, can contribute to health and vitality.

How much do we know today that will help us achieve these goals? Some, but not nearly enough. Intensive research into nutrition and aging is very recent, although a number of theories have historical roots. The Human Nutrition Research Center on Aging is the only one of its kind in this country, probably in the world, and it is only 10 years old! The current edition of the Recommended Dietary Allowances (RDA) includes only two age categories of adults: up to the age of 51, and 51 and above. Not only does such a categorization fail to recognize the remarkable differences between a 55-year-old and an 85-year-old, but in fact the data are based almost entirely on studies of young, healthy individuals. The 10th edition, released in 1989, adds additional age-group categories, but is not based on significantly new information that focuses on the real needs of the elderly. The next edition of the RDA, which probably will appear in 1994, will be the first edition to incorporate information and concepts from studies in the elderly population. Studies of the following issues will be important:

- Energy requirements decline as the muscle mass of an aging person decreases. In turn, fewer calories are used in physical activity. We know, however, that the decline in muscle mass is not inevitable; older people can build muscle with exercise and maintain muscle and skeletal mass by exercise, even if at an efficiency slightly lower than that of young people with regard to the use of protein from the diet.
- A protein intake that may be required to maintain balance in an elderly person may be too high if kidney function is declining. We may also have to adjust protein allowances in such cases.
- The same vitamin A intake in young and elderly people results in very different blood levels of vitamin A and vitamin A esters, because the peripheral tissues of older persons take up the vitamin at much slower rates. It is therefore easier to create higher blood levels of vitamin A in the elderly and, theoretically, easier to produce toxicity.
- The aging process itself may involve oxidation of body tissues. Such a process might call for increased amounts of antioxidant nutrients, such as vitamin E and ascorbic acid, to retard some kinds of degenerative changes.
- Preliminary data from work at Tufts University indicate that some forms of cataracts can be slowed in animals by increasing vitamin C intake. Could this be true in man?
- The decline in immune function with age is retarded by vitamin E. Will this have a place in our future discussion of recommended allowances?
- Preliminary data indicate that, at least for the population among postmenopausal women with the lowest calcium intakes, increasing calcium intake can retard the bone loss that leads to osteoporosis. Should we change our calcium intake targets in postmenopausal women, or in younger

women as well, and what recommendation should we make for exercise, which seems the most reliable way to maintain bone density and health? Should we, for example, have different calcium and protein as well as energy intake standards for the elderly who are more vigorous and who exercise regularly? Because exercise increases intake of vitamins along with calories, should we include exercise as a part of the RDA?

- Depletion of vitamin B_6 results in changes in brain function in the elderly that are much more profound than those in younger people.
- One-third of those over the age of 70 lose their ability to secrete stomach acid, which in turn influences the absorption of nutrients such as iron, folic acid, and calcium. How do we provide for that population?

Nutritional Status of Older People

How well are we doing with diet and nutritional status in the elderly population in this country? The Health and Nutrition Examination Surveys (HANES) of the 1970s and 1980s began to answer some of the questions of nutritional status of the elderly; the next survey, HANES III, will focus on the elderly even more. These and other surveys show that many older people are consuming diets that fail to meet the recommended allowances. Yet few of these individuals show clinical or biochemical signs of nutritional deficiency. Of course, the nutritional status of the population of elders depends upon where you look. We find more anemia, protein malnutrition, and vitamin deficiency in urban, minority populations at a low socioeconomic level. The relationship between poverty and undernutrition, however, has shifted in this country over the last 20 years. Since the White House Conference on Food, Nutrition and Health in 1969 and the White House Conference on Aging in 1971, we have instituted a number of programs that have benefited the elderly in both their economic and nutritional status.

In 1973, in response to the growing population of older Americans, to rising health-care costs, and to greater interest in preventive health care, the Nutrition Program for the Elderly was established as a part of the Administration on Aging. The program expanded food and nutrition services from the hospital to communities and homes. Current Federal programs support the functional independence of older individuals in ambulatory care centers, adult day-care centers, hospices, and home settings. These food and nutrition activities include the USDA Food Stamp Program, which serves more than 2 million older Americans, and two programs administered by the Nutrition Program for Older Americans: Congregate Meals, which also serves about 2 million individuals, and Home-Delivered Meals, which serves 0.5 million. Despite limitations in size, and scope, these programs have improved demonstrably the dietary intake and nutritional status of participants.

Although we cannot be complacent about the access of vigorous, independent elderly people to food, we must continue to focus on the problems of lonely, homebound, economically deprived older people. There will be major differences both in the mechanics of delivering food to this diverse population and in the very nature of the foods.

Current Nutrition Recommendations for Older Adults

The Surgeon General recommends that older Americans consume sufficient nutrients and energy and achieve levels of physical activity that maintain desirable body weight and may prevent or delay the onset of chronic disease. Because it is often difficult to maintain adequate nutrient intake on low-calorie diets, older people should be advised to maintain at least moderate levels of physical activity to increase caloric needs. Recommendations to the general population about calcium intake are also true for older Americans. Because many of the chronic diseases common to older people may originate earlier in life, dietary guidance should be provided consistently throughout life. Sedentary older individuals should be counseled on methods appropriate to increase caloric expenditure. Older persons who do not (or cannot) consume adequate levels of nutrients from food sources and those who have dietary, biochemical, or clinical evidence of inadequate intake should receive advice about the proper type and dosage of nutrient supplements. Such supplements may be appropriate for some older people, but self-prescribed supplementation, especially in large doses, may be harmful and should be discouraged. Older people who suffer from diet-related chronic diseases should receive dietary counseling from dietitians, and those who take medications should be given professional advice on diets that minimize food-drug interactions.

Recommendations for Institutions That Serve Older Adults

Information provided on food labels should be scientifically sound, understandable, and non-misleading. Food services, especially those receiving government funds, should be required to pay special attention to meeting the caloric and nutrient needs of older clients. Nutritional assessment and guidance should be undertaken at hospital admission or at enrollment in or discharge from institutional or community-based services for older adults (for example, acute- and long-term care inpatient services, hospital-based outpatient services, alcohol and drug treatment programs, community health services, and home-delivered meals programs).

Recommendations for Food Industries That Serve Older Adults

Evidence suggests that older people would benefit from food products that provide a high proportion of available nutrients to calories, have taste appeal, and are easy to prepare. Older people who are homebound, live in isolation, or suffer from chronic disease have special needs for foods and nutrition services that are tailored to their particular conditions.

Future Research Priorities

Research on nutrition and aging is currently focused on two major areas: the nutritional requirements and status of aging people and the influence of diet on aging processes and related illnesses. The Surgeon General's report discusses the role of nutrition in the aged. Future research and surveillance issues of special priority in the report include:

- The nutrient and energy requirements of older adults
- The effects of dietary restriction or overconsumption on longevity and age-related illnesses
- The interactions of older Americans among nutritional status, lifestyle, and behavior, and the environment
- The effects of nutrition on age-related impairment of the cardiovascular, gastrointestinal/oral, immune, musculoskeletal, and nervous-system functions and on prevention and treatment of disorders of those systems
- The effects of marginal nutrient and energy deficiencies on the mental and physical health of older people
- Interactions among nutrients and between nutrients and drugs in older adults
- Development of data bases for use by pharmacists and dietitians in counseling older people about drug-nutrient interactions
- Age-specific methods and standards to assess nutritional status and body composition of older adults
- The educational methods and program strategies that best promote adequate food consumption by older persons
- Improved methods to monitor the nutritional status of older populations and individuals, including older adults who have been institutionalized
- The educational and public health strategies that can be used to eliminate nutrition-related health fraud directed toward older citizens

Suggested Reading

Bortz WM, II. Disuse and aging. JAMA 1982;248:1203.

Fiatarone MA, Marks EC, Ryan ND, Meredith CN, Lipsitz LA, Evans WJ. High-intensity strength training in nonagenarians. JAMA 1990;263: 3029-34.

McGandy RB, Russell RM, Hartz SC, Jacob RA, Peters H, Sahyoun N. Nutritional Status Survey of healthy non-institutionalized elderly: nutrient intakes from three-day diet records and nutrient supplements. Nutr Res 1986;6:785-98.

Meredith CN, Zackin MJ, Frontera WR, Evans WJ. Dietary protein requirements and body protein metabolism in endurance-trained men. J Appl Physiol 1989;66(6):2850-6.

Munro HN, McGandy RB, Hartz SC, Russell RM, Jacob RA, Otradovec CL. Protein nutriture of a group of free-living elderly. Am J Clin Nutr 1987;6:586-92.

Shock NW. Some physiological aspects of aging in man. Bull NY Acad Med 1956;32:268-78.

Webb AR, Kline L, Holick MF. Influence of season and latitude on the cutaneous synthesis of vitamin D_3: exposure to winter sunlight in Boston and Edmonton will not promote vitamin D_3 synthesis in human skin. J Clin Endocrinol Metab 1988;61:373-8.

Zheng JJ, Rosenberg IH. What is the nutritional status of the elderly? Geriatrics 1989;44(6):57-64.

5

Taste and Smell: Their Role in Aging and Obesity

SUSAN S. SCHIFFMAN, Ph.D.*

Physiology and Anatomy of Taste and Smell

To understand how the senses of taste and smell operate in obese and elderly people, it is helpful to know something about the physiology and anatomy of these chemical sensing systems. The sense of taste is mediated by taste buds (Figure 1) located on *papillae* in the mouth and throat. If you touch your tongue, you will feel the papillae, which are small protrusions that cover the top surface. Taste buds look like oranges, with small segments called taste cells. There are approximately 50 cells in a taste bud, and the cells are hooked together and can communicate with one another through small connections called *gap junctions*.

*Duke University Medical Center, Durham, North Carolina.

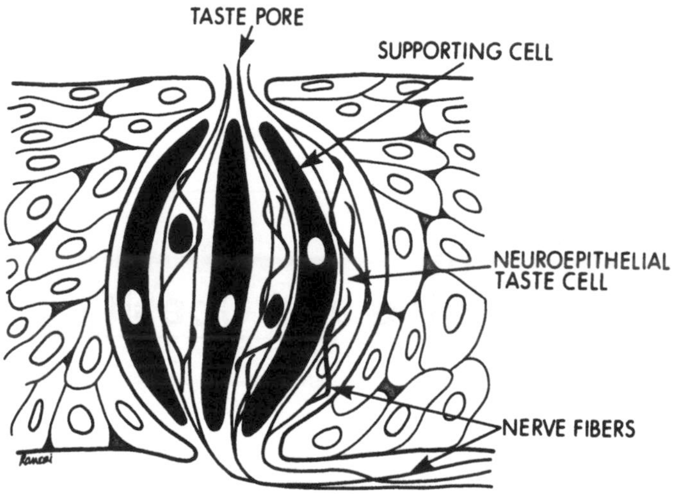

Figure 1 Schematic diagram of a taste bud, which is made up of clusters of taste cells.

Taste cells are formed in the epithelium around the bud and are replaced about every 10 days. This renewal process can be affected by age, disease, drugs, nutritional and hormonal states, therapeutic radiation, and other conditions that interfere with mitosis, or normal cell division. When you burn your tongue with hot food or drink, it takes a few days for taste to return because new taste cells need to be formed to replace the damaged ones. During the aging process, the number of buds and papillae tends to decline. However, it now is believed that decreases in taste perception that occur during aging are related more to losses of receptors at the membrane of the taste cells than to a reduced number of taste cells.

The receptors for smell are bipolar neurons located in the upper portion of the nose (Figure 2). Olfactory receptors, like taste receptors are constantly being replaced, but the average lifespan of an olfactory cell is 30 days. The olfactory receptor neurons course through a small bone, the *cribriform plate*, into the olfactory bulbs located under the anterior portion of the brain (Figure 3). In the olfactory

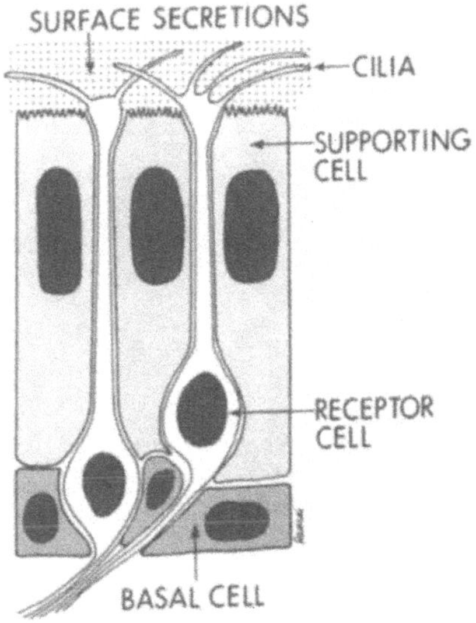

Figure 2 Schematic diagram of the olfactory epithelium that shows receptor cells along with supporting and basal cells.

bulbs there are groups of cells called *glomeruli*. With age many glomeruli are lost, and the bulb actually looks moth-eaten. Cells in the olfactory bulb project to areas of the brain that are responsible for our emotions. Thus, the parts of the brain that control emotions and olfaction overlap anatomically. These areas, which are called the "*old brain*" and consist of the hippocampus, amygdala, and prepyriform cortex, are especially vulnerable to aging. Neurons in these areas exhibit the first degeneration in the aging brain.

The sense of smell is generally the first sensory system to fail with age. There are several reasons for its vulnerability. First, viruses and pollutants can be transported from the nose up the olfactory pathways into the brain, where they cause direct damage. One theory to explain the development of Alzheimer's disease, a dementing illness of old age, is that it begins in the nose as a result of breathing aluminosilicates which are transported into the hippocampus, amygdala, and prepyriform cortex. Pollutants such as aluminosilicates

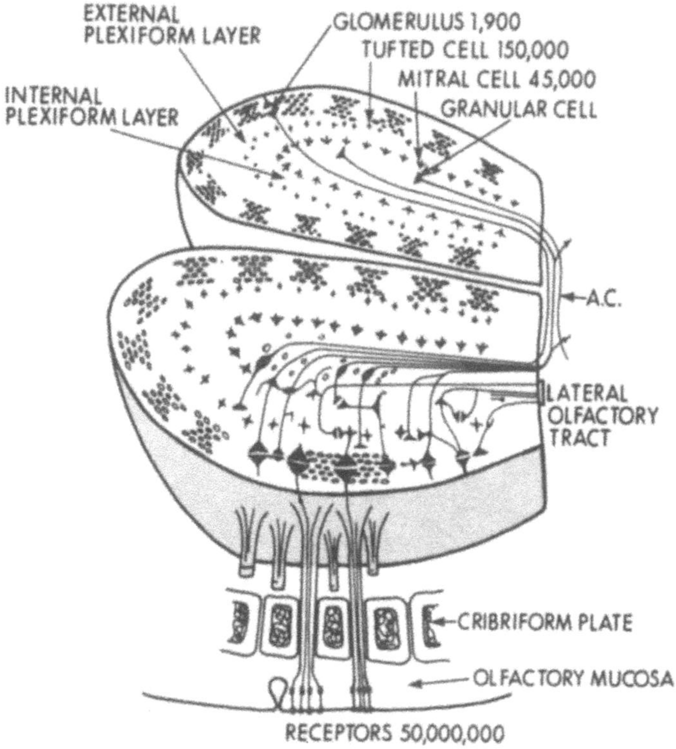

Figure 3 Schematic diagram of cross-section of the olfactory bulb.

may be responsible for the development of neurofibrillary tangles and senile plaques that invade these brain areas even in normal aging; such tangles and plaques are found in abundance in Alzheimer's disease. Second, the "old brain" was the first cortex to evolve; it is architecturally different from the cortical areas that evolved later and are less vulnerable to attack.

Chemosensory Losses with Age

Perceptual losses in the senses of taste and smell accompany the aging process. Chemosensory losses are usually classified in the following way: *ageusia* (absence of taste), *hypogeusia* (diminished taste), *dysgeusia* (distortion of normal taste), *anosmia* (absence of smell), *hyposmia* (diminished sensitivity of smell), and *dysosmia* (distortion of normal smell). The perceptual losses that occur in each of these conditions result not only from anatomical losses associated with normal aging but also from some diseases, pharmacological and surgical interventions, radiation, and environmental pollutants.

The reduced taste and smell acuity in elderly patients can contribute to anorexia, weight loss, and malnutrition. For this reason it is important to find practical measures for the treatment of chemosensory losses. In the United States in 1980, 15.7% of the population was more than 60 years old, and chemosensory research studies suggest that the majority of this group has some loss of taste or smell. By the year 2030, 20% of Americans (50 million people) will be over the age of 65.

Perceptual Loss in Taste

Losses in taste sensitivity have been reported consistently in the elderly, but such losses are not nearly as great as losses in olfaction. On the average, taste thresholds for amino acids, sweeteners, and sodium chloride are 2 to 2.5 times higher in people over 65 years old when compared with the young. However, thresholds that are over 20 times higher for the elderly have been reported for sodium citrate, sodium tartrate, and sodium sulfate.

The increased thresholds for amino acids in older individuals can be advantageous, because foods that are nutritionally fortified with bitter-tasting amino acids such as methionine are not objectionable. However, increased thresholds for salt and sugar are clearly a disadvantage. Increased sweet thresholds can expose the elderly to any adverse effects that result from ingesting sugar or sodium saccharin. Sensory losses for the salty taste can lead to increased use of salt and difficulty in complying with a physician's recommendation of a low-salt diet.

The perceived intensity for suprathreshold tastants also diminishes with age. Suprathreshold losses for the tastes of two amino acids (glutamic acid and aspartic acid) are relatively larger than for other amino acids. This is noteworthy because reduced glutamate binding has recently been implicated in Alzheimer's disease. Identification tasks also reveal that the ability to recognize common tastes as well as foods is diminished in old age. These losses can result not only from normal aging but also from other causes, including diseases and drugs.

Perceptual Losses of Smell

There is a broad general decline in olfactory functioning with age. Elevated detection and recognition thresholds have been reported for a wide range of odors including foods, purified odorants, and coal gas. Odor-detection thresholds for a range of food flavors including cherry, grape, and lemon are at least 11 times higher on average for the elderly when compared with the young. Sensitivity to other compounds such as steroids that have urine-like odors is also reduced in the elderly. The diminished sensitivity to food odors is a distinct disadvantage and can result in reduced appreciation of food and even lead to malnutrition.

The losses in olfactory sensitivity generally begin in the 60s and become more severe in persons who are more than 70 years old. For example, people in their 60s often have great difficulty identifying different varieties of coffee or brands of beer on the basis of odor and taste. Losses can occur in the 40s and 50s for a small portion of the population. These losses result from a variety of causes, including normal aging, disease, and drugs.

Odor and Taste Enhancement for Treating Age-Related Chemosensory Losses

Odor Enhancement

The addition of commercial flavors to foods for the elderly has been a practical means of improving food intake and subsequent nutritional status. It has been used extensively in both hospital and nursing-home settings to increase intake of nutrient-dense foods in older people.

Taste Enhancement

Research on the enhancement properties of chemicals ultimately may be useful in treating taste losses that occur with old age. Studies of taste transduction and modulation mechanisms have found four pharmacological agents that enhance taste perception: caffeine (and other methyl xanthines), 5′-nucleotides, inosine, and bretylium tosylate. Although several of these agents are not practical taste enhancers, they do give some insight into the means by which taste sensations can be amplified.

Methyl Xanthines

Methyl xanthines are compounds found in coffee, tea, and chocolate and include caffeine, theophylline, and theobromine. Methyl xanthines exert their effect by blocking adenosine receptors. Adenosine controls and regulates a variety of biological processes; for example, it slows sinus rate and leads to atrioventricular block, vasodilation, and hypotension. Methyl xanthines can bind to adenosine receptors and antagonize the effects of adenosine. In taste experiments, caffeine and other methyl xanthines have been found to enhance taste by blocking adenosine receptors. For example, application of low concentrations of caffeine (10 μM to 10 mM) to the anterior tongue for 4 minutes enhances the taste of artificial sweeteners that have bitter components, including sodium saccharin. Caffeine also slightly enhances the tastes of table salt (NaCl) and the salt substitute KCl. However, the taste of sweeteners without bitter components, such as sucrose and aspartame, is not enhanced by methyl xanthines. Methyl xanthines are believed to enhance taste by increasing a compound called cAMP (cyclic adenosine monophosphate) inside cells.

5′-Ribonucleotides

Researchers have known for some time that 5′-ribonucleotides, including inosine-5′-monophosphate (IMP) and guanosine-5′-monophosphate (GMP), enhance the taste of monosodium glutamate. Recently, it has been shown that application of 1 mM IMP to the tongue also enhances the sweet taste of aspartame and sucrose. Sweeteners such as calcium cyclamate and sodium saccharin that have bitter components, however, and other substances that have salty, sour, or bitter tastes are unaffected by adaptation to IMP.

Inosine

Inosine is a breakdown product of both IMP and adenosine. Application of inosine to the tongue enhances the tastes of sucrose, aspartame, and sodium saccharin. It has no potentiating effect on any sweetener enhanced by caffeine.

Bretylium Tosylate

Bretylium tosylate is a compound that contains a positively charged nitrogen atom. When applied to the tongue for 4 minutes, it enhances the salt taste for both humans and rats. Although the mechanism of this enhancement is not known, it may act by opening channels in the taste cell membrane that permit an influx of Na^+ into the taste cell.

Practical Limitations of Taste Enhancers

Caffeine, inosine, and bretylium tosylate require a 4-minute application period. Caffeine and other methyl xanthines have central pharmacological effects. IMP has been used to potentiate the glutamate taste, but little is known about long-term usage at higher levels. Inosine has never been used as an enhancer, and bretylium tosylate is an antifibrillary drug and will never be used in food. Despite these problems, the use of these pharmacological probes has provided insight into the biochemical properties that ultimately must be invoked by practical taste enhancers.

Texture Enhancement

The addition of texture to foods (crunch, chewiness) can partially compensate for loss of odor and taste sensitivity. However, this strategy is appropriate only for elderly people without problems of dentition. For persons with tooth loss, dental caries, and periodontal disease, softer textured foods with added functional fiber and flavors should be designed. Addition of ingredients that stimulate salivation may also be helpful for older people taking medications that reduce salivation.

Taste and Smell in Obesity

Psychophysical studies of taste and smell perception reveal that there are no significant differences in absolute sensitivity to chemosensory stimuli between obese and thin individuals. Threshold and intensity measures that evaluate the ability to perceive chemosensory stimuli do not differ with body weight. However, there are significant differences in taste and smell preferences in obese and thin persons. Overweight people prefer a diet that has a greater sensory impact and variety than their thinner counterparts. Each of us, whether thin or overweight, has a "set point" for flavor and texture. Our set point is the amount of sensation we require from our food and beverages to feel satisfied with what we have eaten.

An elevated flavor and texture set point has several causes. First, it can be caused by the experience of dieting itself. Flavor and texture deprivation during liquid and other bland diets compounded by exposure to intense and varied foods during a binge can increase the preference for high-flavor foods. Second, the food selections of overweight people have been shown to contain a higher percentage of calories from fat; much of this fat is termed "hidden fat" because it is found in solid form and is not directly visible. Because odorants are predominantly fat-soluble, persons whose diets are high in fat can become acclimated to high flavor levels. In addition, fats convey many of the mechanical and geometric characteristics that are responsible for such food textures as crispness, crunchiness, creaminess, and elasticity. Third, the simple act of eating more, whether for pleasure or to deal with uncomfortable states such as boredom, anger, or stress, accustoms people to greater amounts of flavor. Fourth, people who live in the melting-pot culture of the United States are exposed to textures and flavors from a wider variety of ethnic cuisines (for example, Mexican, Creole, Asian, Cuban) than are people who live in a more homogeneous culture.

The need of the overweight person to have a variety of textures and flavors presents a challenge to the clinician who is trying to achieve weight loss in a patient by means of a low-fat diet. To date, most clinicians have not used diets that take the sensory needs of the obese patient into account; rather, they use traditional treatments for obesity, i.e., liquid and/or bland low-fat diets. The long-term success with these traditional treatments, however, is poor. The failure rate often approaches 97%, because this unappetizing fare does not meet the sensory needs of overweight people. The need for a wide range of tastes and smells is probably part of our biological heritage. Primitive man ate foods with a wide range of tastes and textures: nuts (crunchy), berries (sweet, juicy), fish (flaky), and fowl and venison (chewy).

Two treatment strategies that consider the high flavor-texture set point of the overweight patient have been attempted. One lowers a patient's desire for flavor and texture through hypnosis and behavioral techniques. Unfortunately, this approach has failed dismally with most patients.

Another more successful treatment strategy is to provide high flavor and texture along with a diet low in fat and calories. This approach was first found to be successful in a 2-week clinical study. Three groups of overweight subjects were placed on a diet of 1000 Calories per day for 2 weeks. For the first group, noncaloric flavors were added to the food to amplify the flavor. The second (control) group ate the same foods as the first group but without the additional flavors. The third group ate the same foods as the second group but also used chocolate and vanilla flavor sprays that provided an intense burst of flavor on the tongue. Persons in the third group were instructed to use the sprays whenever they had a craving for sweets. Over the 2 weeks, the average weight loss was 4.61 pounds in the first group and 4.34 pounds in the third group. The second group lost an average of only 3.47 pounds. The losses of the "flavor" groups were significantly greater than those of the control group.

Food preferences of obese individuals may result in part from genetic differences in the way they perceive bitter tastes. Some people can detect the bitter taste in a compound called PTC (phenylthiocarbamide) while others cannot. People who taste the bitterness of PTC tend to dislike bitter-tasting vegetables such as brussels sprouts. In addition, more people who can taste bitterness in PTC also tend to dislike saccharin-sweetened drinks and scotch whiskey than those who cannot, because "tasters" perceive more unpleasant sensory components. Among 90 of my overweight patients, 87% were tasters of PTC; only 74% of an equal number of thin subjects were tasters. It may be that some overweight people avoid low-fat vegetables, which would help them lose weight, because they cannot tolerate the taste.

Suggested Reading

Schiffman SS. Changes in taste and smell with age: psychophysical aspects. In: Ordy JM, Brizzee K, eds. Sensory Systems and Communication in the Elderly. Aging, Vol 10. New York: Raven Press, 1979:227-46.

Schiffman SS, Orlandi M, Erickson RP. Changes in taste and smell with age: biological aspects. In: Ordy JM, Brizzee K, eds. Sensory Systems and Communication in the Elderly. Aging, Vol 10. New York: Raven Press, 1979:247-68.

Schiffman SS. Taste and smell in disease. N Engl J Med 1983;308:1275-9, 1337-43.

Schiffman SS. The nose as a port of entry for aluminosilicates and other pollutants: possible role in Alzheimer's disease. Neurobiol Aging 1986;7:576-8.

Schiffman SS. The use of flavor to enhance efficacy of reducing diets. Hosp Pract 1986;21:44H,K,N,P,R.

Schiffman SS. Smell. In: Maddox GL, ed. Encyclopedia of Aging. New York: Springer, 1987:618-9.

Schiffman SS. Taste. In: Maddox GL, ed. Encyclopedia of Aging. New York: Springer, 1987:655-8.

Schiffman SS. Recent developments in taste enhancement. Food Technol 1987;41:72-3,124.

Schiffman SS, Warwick ZS. Flavor enhancement of foods for the elderly can reverse anorexia. Neurobiol Aging 1988;9:24-6.

6

Determinants of Food Intake and Selection

BARBARA J. ROLLS, Ph.D.*

Introduction

You are in a supermarket surrounded by food. How do you decide which foods to buy? Your decision may be based on the perceived healthfulness or the cost of the food, or perhaps on the influence of a clever advertisement. Although food choices are a result of many influences, research shows that taste is the major determinant. We buy the foods that we or our families like to eat. How, then, do we learn to like particular foods?

Rozin has described three types of influences on food selection. Biological and genetic influences, such as an innate preference for

*Laboratory for the Study of Human Ingestive Behavior, Johns Hopkins University, Baltimore, Maryland.

sweetness, are the first. Genetic influences fall into this category, although evidence from twin studies offers little support, in that identical twins have no more similar preferences than fraternal twins. Some evidence does indicate that food choices can be influenced by hormones or by the need for particular nutrients. Cultural background is the second, and the most important, of the three influences on food selection. According to Rozin, other influences are minor when compared with that of cultural background. The third influence is the unique set of food experiences that contributes to a specific pattern of food likes and dislikes in each person. For example, we learn to avoid foods that make us ill and to consume foods that satisfy our hunger.

Studies conducted by Davis in the 1920s examined the development of food preferences in early life. She studied newly weaned infants who self-selected their diets from an array of nutritious foods. During the first few weeks of the study, the infants tasted all the foods and even the plates and cutlery. Gradually, distinct likes and dislikes emerged. The general pattern of consumption included three solid foods at a meal. Although the infants had favorite foods, they nonetheless ate varied meals. In the short term, meals were not always balanced, but over longer periods, the children consumed foods appropriate for their nutritional needs, remained healthy, and grew normally. Davis concluded that some innate, automatic mechanism exists in infants that helps ensure good nutrition.

Mechanisms That Influence Food Intake

Our research has shown why humans tend to eat a variety of foods. Food preferences vary not only among different persons, but also within a given person. Palatability, or the pleasantness of a food's taste, is not constant and can change as a food is being consumed. We have studied the changing response to foods in a series of laboratory experiments. Although a laboratory is an unnatural setting, its use affords us sufficient control to isolate specific influences on eating behavior.

I will briefly describe our experimental protocols for food intake. We usually schedule subjects to arrive at the laboratory at lunchtime, so they will be moderately hungry. They have not been told the purpose of the experiment, because that knowledge might alter their behavior. The subjects first taste, then rate their preference for, a number of different foods. Subjective feelings about hunger and the taste of foods are assessed using visual analog scales. After rating their fullness and the taste of specific foods, each subject receives a test meal of a food he or she has just rated. Subjects are instructed to eat as much of the food as they wish. When they have finished eating, they again assess their hunger and the taste of the foods sampled before the test meal. We can then determine what effect the consumption of a test meal had on the pleasantness of the taste of other foods.

We have found that satiety, or the feeling of having had enough to eat, is specific to a particular food that has been consumed. If, for example, chocolates are eaten until a subject feels full, the pleassantness of the taste, smell, appearance, and texture of chocolates will have declined. The subject also finds, however, that the pleasantness of the sensory properties of other foods, particularly those very different from chocolates, will not have declined at all. The changes in pleasantness relate directly to the amounts of various foods that will be eaten during a meal: One may have eaten enough of a particular food and that food will no longer be appealing, but the appetite for other foods will remain. We call these changes "sensory-specific satiety," and such changes help ensure that a variety of foods will be consumed in a meal. The changing response to foods *as they are consumed* is probably the key to the consumption of a balanced diet by the infants in the Davis study.

Sensory-specific satiety, or the changes in the palatability of foods that occur while the foods are being eaten, can affect food intake and selection. What is it about foods, then, that makes us like them less after we have eaten them? We have investigated the following explanations:

1. *The changes in palatability occur as a result of particular nutrients in the food eaten*. For example, after a large amount of a high-fat food has been consumed, other high-fat foods are not appealing. We have been unable to find experimental support for this hypothesis.

2. *Decreased palatability is a response to the calories in the food eaten*. That is, the pleasantness of the taste of foods depends on a physiological need for calories. We have sweetened foods with aspartame to test the role of calories in sensory-specific satiety; we found no difference in the effect on palatability whether the desserts were sweetened with aspartame or sucrose. Our results in this study do not support the hypothesis.

3. *Decreased palatability results from tiring of the particular sensory characteristics of foods as they are eaten*. For example, after a large amount of a sweet food has been eaten, the tendency is to dislike other sweet foods, regardless of the nutrient content or energy density of the foods. Salty foods, however, are still appetizing. Particular types of foods also lose their appeal; for example, if one kind of soup has been served, other soups are not appetizing. Thus, the desire for variety during a meal appears to be a desire for different sensory experiences. Our experimental results tend to support this explanation for changes in food palatability.

The provision of a wide variety of foods may ensure that a balance of nutrients is consumed. If, however, satiety, i.e., the termination of eating, is specific to a food that has been eaten, overeating may occur in response to a wide variety of readily available foods.

We have studied the effects of variety in a meal on food intake. When we offered a four-course meal of very different foods—sausages, bread and butter, chocolate dessert, and bananas—food intake was 60% higher than when a meal consisted of only one of those foods. The results indicate that caloric intake is not regulated precisely during the course of a single meal.

We have also found that the greater the difference among the sensory properties of the various foods in a meal, the greater the enhancement of food intake. In the study just discussed, the availability of four very different foods increased intake by 60%. Similar foods, such as sandwiches with four different fillings, increased intake by 33%. Three different flavors of yogurt, which also differed in appearance and texture, increased intake by 20%. Even as simple a variation as a meal of three different pasta shapes increased intake by 15% compared to the intake of a meal with only the favorite pasta shape.

Our studies indicate, therefore, that if one wishes to increase appetite or encourage eating, the available foods should be as varied as possible; if the aim is to decrease appetite or to keep food intake low, the variety of available foods should be kept to the minimum necessary for a balanced diet.

Our studies also emphasize that food intake is not regulated precisely in the short term, that is, during a meal. Intake is affected not only by palatability but also by other factors, such as stress and social situation. For example, de Castro and de Castro have recently shown that we eat more when eating with others than when eating alone. Nevertheless, some studies show that humans do have the ability to adjust caloric intake to meet energy demands. In the 1970s, Fomon studied the food intake of bottle-fed infants whose formulas varied in the amount of calories. He found that after approximately 40 days of age, the infants adjusted the volume of formula they drank to maintain a constant daily caloric intake.

Aspartame and Food Intake

The standard method with which to test the regulation of caloric intake in adults is to give a fixed amount of various foods, then determine how much food is eaten subsequently. In many of these "preloading" studies, aspartame has been used to vary the calories in the preload meal. The studies have enabled us to examine not only the ability of humans to regulate their caloric intake, but also the effects of aspartame consumption on hunger and food intake.

Replacing the sugar in foods or drinks with a low-energy sweetener will lead to a reduction in caloric intake if the diets of the consumers are otherwise unchanged. It has been suggested, however, that intense sweeteners such as aspartame and saccharin may increase appetite and food intake and therefore may be without benefit in weight control or, worse, may lead to weight gain.

A controversy began in 1986 when Blundell and Hill published a letter in *The Lancet*, titled "Paradoxical effects of an intense sweetener (aspartame) on appetite." Shortly thereafter, Tordoff and Friedman at the Monell Chemical Senses Center claimed that saccharin increased food intake in rats. Much work has been done on the effects of sweeteners on appetite and food intake in humans, and it seems appropriate to summarize the results of these studies.

Blundell and Hill found that a solution of aspartame decreased the pleasantness of the sweet taste, although not as effectively as in our studies. (We found both aspartame- and sucrose-sweetened gelatin desserts equally effective in decreasing the pleasantness of the sweet taste.) The paradox referred to by Blundell and Hill in the title of their study is that, although the pleasantness of the sweet taste was reduced, hunger not only was not reduced, but was in fact sometimes increased after the preload. Their results, however, raise questions about methodological issues, the most important of which is that ratings of hunger do not necessarily relate to actual food consumption. It is imperative, therefore, that such studies include measures of food intake. Since their first report, Blundell and his colleagues have measured food intake after ingestion of drinks, foods, or capsules containing aspartame. Their new studies have not found increases in food intake, and they have sometimes shown decreases. They did report that yogurt sweetened with saccharin increased food intake.

During the past two years, several reports from other groups have indicated that aspartame in foods and drinks increases neither hunger nor food intake. Recently, our laboratory has also conducted several studies using aspartame. One of the studies examined the effects of consuming commercially available pudding and gelatin desserts sweetened with either aspartame or sucrose on subjective appetite ratings of food intake. When normal-weight, nondieting men and women were given large portions of either a low- or high-calorie pudding or gelatin dessert and instructed to eat as much as they liked, they ate similar weights of the different caloric versions of each food. Despite the resulting differences in caloric intake (up to 200 kcal), food intake of subjects did not show a statistically significant trend toward caloric compensation when a variety of foods was presented 2 hours later. Total caloric intake (preload plus test meal) did not differ between groups. Ratings of hunger, desire to eat, the amount subjects wanted to eat, and the pleasantness of the consumed food were similarly decreased and fullness similarly increased by consumption of either the low- or high-caloric version of the foods. Awareness of the caloric content of the foods did not influence intake or appetite; both informed and uninformed subjects responded similarly in the tests. Thus, reduced-calorie foods sweetened with aspartame suppressed ratings of hunger for several hours after consumption.

We have just completed a study that compares the effects of aspartame- and sucrose-sweetened lemonades. The study was designed to test whether the differences between our findings and those of Blundell were based on our use of solid foods versus his use of solutions. Our subjects could not tell which sweetener was used in the lemonade. We conducted three studies with seven different conditions: Subjects consumed 8 or 16 ounces of aspartame- or sucrose-sweetened lemonade or plain water or no drink, either with a self-selected lunch or 30 or 60 minutes before the lunch. When drinks were taken with the meal, we found that more calories (lunch plus drinks) were consumed when subjects received sucrose-sweetened drinks. Thus, diet drinks taken with a meal can aid in reducing caloric intake. We saw no indication that aspartame increased ratings of hunger. We also found that sucrose-sweetened drinks taken with the meal satisfied thirst less well than either aspartame-sweetened drinks or plain water.

Most recent studies have failed to show an increase in appetite or food intake with aspartame, and the controversy has therefore diminished. One notable exception is the study by Tordoff and Alleva at the Monell Chemical Senses Center. They found that chewing gum sweetened with some concentrations of aspartame increased reported hunger. They did not, however, determine whether food intake was affected, which is a critical part of such studies. It is noteworthy that these same workers recently reported that consumption of soda sweetened with aspartame resulted in reduced caloric intake and weight loss over three weeks, while consumption of soda sweetened with high-fructose corn syrup had the opposite effect, i.e., increased caloric intake and weight gain.

This study is particularly relevant because it measured intake over several weeks. One might argue that an examination of intake during a single meal does not indicate what will happen from meal to meal. Although intake may vary widely in a meal, regulation is believed to be more precise over longer periods. We make this assumption in part because may people maintain a fairly constant body weight. If one considers that each of us eats approximately one ton of food per year in more than 1000 meals, and that an error of only 2% would lead to a weight gain of 80 pounds in 20 years, it seems likely that food intake is regulated. Several years ago, Garrow in London provocatively suggested that no clear evidence exists to show that humans possess an intrinsic mechanism to regulate food intake. He suggested instead that body weight was maintained at a constant level by external cues, such as the bathroom scales or the fit of clothing. Other scientists have suggested that regulation of food intake is not that important because excess energy can be eliminated by increasing whole-body energy expenditure.

It is now clear that the mechanisms that rid us of excess energy cannot adequately balance large deviations in energy intake. To determine whether there are mechanisms that detect the energy needs of the body and translate this information into appropriate food intake, studies have been conducted in which the energy content of the diet was altered over several days or weeks. The studies then examined whether the calorie-intake level remained constant during such a challenge; a constant caloric intake would indicate the presence of a regulatory mechanism.

Highly controlled studies in which aspartame replaced sugar were conducted by Porikos and her colleagues. Normal-weight and obese subjects were confined to a hospital room for the duration of the study. Foods were served from platters, and subjects, who were not aware that intake was being measured, helped themselves. Subjects were required to drink at least two sodas per day. During the first six days of the test, the foods and drinks were sweetened with sucrose. The free availability of a variety of foods led both obese and normal-weight subjects to gain weight during this period. On day 7, the sucrose was replaced with aspartame, which resulted in a 25% decrease in energy intake. For the first several days of the aspartame regimen, subjects continued to eat the same weight of food that they had consumed during the sucrose regimen. After several days, the subjects consumed more food to compensate for some of the missing calories, but daily caloric intake remained significantly (approximately 15%) below baseline levels. The weight gain observed during the baseline period stopped, and weight stayed constant. Subjects in this study were required to consume some reduced calorie sodas, and the available sweet foods all had reduced calories, so it is possible that subjects could not have consumed enough food to compensate for the missing calories.

Fat and Food Intake

In other long-term studies, the dietary content of fat or fat and carbohydrate has been manipulated. Studies of dietary fat hold more interest than those of sugar, because sugar makes up approximately 10% of the average American diet, whereas fat contributes approximately 40%. Dietary fat also poses a greater health threat and a greater challenge to the regulation of body weight.

We have recently conducted an experiment in which we surreptitiously manipulated either the fat or carbohydrate content of lunch by 400 kcal (approximately 15% of the daily caloric intake). The subjects were six, normal-weight, nondieting men who lived in a residential laboratory in which food intake could be measured accurately. Apart from the required lunch, subjects could select freely from a wide variety of foods. The subjects accurately compensated for the reduction in calories and maintained a constant energy intake throughout the 13 days of the experiment. We found no statistically significant differences between responses to a reduction in fat compared with that in carbohydrate. The compensation took place within 5 hours of the manipulation, i.e., at dinner, and was observed on the first day of the 3-day manipulation period. Although caloric intake was constant, the intake of various macronutrients was affected by the content of the lunches. The highest fat intake, for example, occurred when subjects ate a high-fat lunch.

Other studies in which the fat content of the diet was manipulated indicate that if enough low-fat foods are available throughout the day, both caloric and fat intake are reduced. As in the aspartame studies, situations can be created in which the amount of food required to make up the caloric deficit is so large that subjects cannot adjust intake. If only a few foods are low-fat, however, and a variety of palatable foods is readily available, compensation for the caloric reduction will probably occur, but will probably be accompanied by a reduction in fat intake.

Fat substitutes may become widely available. Thus, it is important to investigate further their effect on total caloric intake and nutrient balance. The studies reviewed in the present report indicate that caloric intake during a single meal is not tightly regulated, but daily caloric intake can be well regulated. Because intake of individual nutrients does not appear to be tightly controlled, fat substitutes may be beneficial in reducing the percentage of calories from fat in the diet.

It is clear that food selection and intake are affected by a number of different factors that are just beginning to be understood. New developments in food technology, such as sugar and fat substitutes, will enable much larger surreptitious caloric manipulations than have previously been possible. Such studies will increase our understanding of how the intake of calories and nutrients is regulated not only during a meal, but over longer periods.

Suggested Reading

Anderson GH, Saravis S, Schacher R, Zlotkin S, Leiter L. Aspartame: effect on lunch-time food intake, appetite, and hedonic response in children. Appetite 1989;13:93-103.

Birch LL, McPhee L, Sullivan S. Children's food intake following drinks sweetened with sucrose or aspartame: time course effects. Physiol Behav 1989;45:387-95.

Blundell JE, Hill AJ. Paradoxical effects of an intense sweetener (aspartame) on appetite. Lancet 1986;1:1092.

Davis CM. Self selection of diet by newly weaned infants. Am J Dis Child 1928;36:651-79.

de Castro JM, de Castro ES. Spontaneous meal patterns of humans: influence of the presence of other people. Am J Clin Nutr 1989;50:237-47.

Foltin RW, Fischman MW, Moran TH, Rolls BJ, Kelly TH. Caloric compensation for lunches varying in fat and carbohydrate content by humans in a residential laboratory. Am J Clin Nutr 1990;52:969-90.

Fomon SJ. Infant Nutrition. Philadelphia: Saunders, 1974.

Lissner L, Levitsky DA, Strupp BJ, Kalkwarf HJ, Roe DA. Dietary fat and the regulation of energy intake in human subjects. Am J Clin Nutr 1987;30:1638-44.

Porikos KP, Hesser MF, Van Itallic TB. Caloric regulation in normal weight men maintained on a palatable diet of conventional foods. Physiol Behav 1982;29:293-300.

Rogers PJ, Blundell JE. Separating the actions of sweetness and calories: effects of saccharin and carbohydrates on hunger and food intake in human subjects. Physiol Behav 1989;45:1093-99.

Rogers PJ, Carlyle J, Hill AJ, Blundell JE. Uncoupling sweet taste and calories: comparison of the effects of glucose and three intense sweeteners on hunger and food intake. 1988;43:547-52.

Rolls BJ. Sensory-specific satiety. Nutr Rev 1986;44:93-101.

Rolls BJ. Effects of intense sweeteners on hunger, food intake and body weight. Am J Clin Nutr; in press.

Rolls BJ, Hetherington M, Burley VJ. The specificity of satiety: the influence of foods of different macronutrient content on the development of satiety. Physiol Behav 1988;43:145-53.

Rolls BJ, Hetherington M, Burley VJ. Sensory stimulation and energy density in the development of satiety. Physiol Behav 1988;44:727-33.

Rolls BJ, Hetherington M, Burley VJ, van Duijvenvoorde PM. Changing hedonic responses to foods during and after a meal. In: Kare MR, Brand JG, eds. Interaction of the Chemical Senses with Nutrition. New York: Academic Press, 1986:247-68.

Rolls BJ, Kim S, Fedoroff IC. Effects of drinks sweetened with sucrose or aspartame on hunger, thirst and food intake in men. Physiol Behav 1990;48:19-26.

Rolls BJ, Laster LJ, Summerfelt A. Hunger and food intake following consumption of low-calorie foods. Appetite 1989;13:115-27.

Rozin P, Vollmecke TA. Food likes and dislikes. Ann Rev Nutr 1986; 6:433-56.

Tordoff MG, Alleva AM. Oral stimulation with aspartame increases hunger. Physiol Behav 1990;47:555-9.

Tordoff MG, Alleva AM. Effect of drinking soda sweetened with aspartame or high-fructose corn syrup on food intake and body weight. Am J Clin Nutr 1990;51:963-9.

Tordoff MG, Friedman MI. Drinking saccharin increases food intake and preference: I. Comparison with other drinks. Appetite 1989;12: 1-10.

7

Technology, Food Safety, and Federal Regulation

SANFORD A. MILLER, Ph.D.*

Introduction

Technology and innovation in the food industry are vital not only to our economy but also to the maintenance and continued improvement of the health of our nation's citizens. The current ability of the United States to compete in global markets, however, is in question. At a recent conference on food research needs in the United States it was observed that "As the U.S. competitive edge erodes on a rising wave of better directed and more adequately supported foreign technologies, we abdicate our own public policy decisions to those external forces." Many people are concerned that this loss of competitiveness will adversely affect the future of the food industry in the United States. As members of industry, academia,

*The University of Texas Health Science Center, San Antonio, Texas.

and government, we must work together to maintain our ability to develop new food technologies and to influence the global economy.

A new food industry has recently developed ingredients that have been specially designed to be components of food that fulfill specific metabolic or manufacturing needs, particularly needs associated with improved health and disease prevention. Despite their potential value, however, designed food components also arouse concerns for public health. Such new substances can make up a substantial portion of a diet; approval for their use, therefore, requires careful consideration of their impact on all segments of the population, from infants to the very elderly.

We do know that chemicals have been added to foods since the advent of human society. Preservation techniques such as salting, smoking, and fermenting have been used for thousands of years; the addition of chemicals to food is not an invention of the modern food industry to poison people or to make money. It is true, however, that many of the ancient food-preservation techniques added (and still add) substances to foods that today are the focus of health-related issues. Over time, the knowledge of methods for the preservation and distribution of food increased. These phenomena in turn enabled the development of cities, and ultimately civilization. Among the new technologies were many that today we consider biotechnologies: brewing, baking, and genetic modification through selection. The ability, first by accident, then by design, to breed animals and plants for increased productivity or resistance to disease was vital to the development of modern society.

Urban cultures expanded to a point at which the food supply became growth-limiting, but the discovery of new technologies for food preservation enabled an expansion of the food supply. These discoveries included canning (thermal processing) in the late 18th century, new chemical additives from the German revolution in organic chemistry in the 19th century, and freezing in the early 20th century.

The increased value of the food supply also led to problems of fraud and adulteration. In 1820 Frederick Accum published *Adulteration of Food*, a seminal book in modern food regulation. This book led to the development of a new scientific field, food analysis. Common food adulterations in the mid-19th century included the addition of acid to whiskey, sand to sugar, alum to flour, and chalk to milk. Accum's book and the public outcry led to the passage in 1845 of England's first food law. It was followed by a stronger English law in 1860 and an American food law in 1906. Interestingly, safety was not an issue in the development of these laws; the emphasis was on adulteration as an economic issue. Food safety was not mentioned in a law in the United States until 1938 (the National Food, Drug and Cosmetic Act), and food safety was not defined legally until 1958. The important part of this story is that science is necessary not only to advance the food industry but also to regulate it.

The first supermarket in the United States was opened in 1938 and contained 670 items. In 1979, the average supermarket contained 12,000 items, and in 1987, modern megamarkets contained as many as 100,000 items. Although most of these products are imitations of one another, some represent the exploitation of major advances in science and technology. Today modern also means mobile. More and more often, food is prepared and consumed away from the home. Modern technology has enabled us to prepare food in one place, preserve it, transport it, and rapidly reheat it.

Ensuring a Safe Food Supply

The food supply is obviously a dynamic entity. Its increasing sophistication enables it to become safer and to feed an almost unlimited number of people, and in the process maintain and improve their health and well-being. At the same time, the sources of our food supply are becoming more and more remote from those of us who consume it. Our grandmothers could determine precisely the origin of the meat or vegetables they consumed and therefore knew the history of the food and whether it was fresh and safe for consumption. Each generation learned the signs that indicated the safety and quality of their food. Today people do not learn these signs because they believe that modern food processing and technology have attended to these problems for them. It has become the government's function to regulate the food industry to ensure that the food supply is safe and of high quality.

The goal of a safe, high-quality food supply, however, has become more difficult to reach. Ensuring food safety or food wholesomeness involves the use of three interrelated disciplines: toxicology, microbiology, and nutrition. The evaluation of new products involves all three.

Toxicology

The problems of chemical safety and toxicology are particularly difficult. A major problem is understanding the significance of increasingly smaller amounts of substances in food. The issues of quantification and determination of the biological meaning of amounts are significant in contemporary food-safety science. Beginning with the 1940s, each decade of the 20th century has produced a new technique enabling the identification of smaller and smaller amounts of a given substance. Today our technical ability to identify such small amounts has far outdistanced our ability to understand the biological significance of such small numbers. Because of these techniques, we can now identify minute amounts of carcinogenic substances (sometimes naturally occurring) in foods that were once thought to be completely "pure." Although our ability to distinguish such small amounts means that we no longer can find "zero" concentrations, we nevertheless operate under a law, the Food, Drug and Cosmetic Act, that mandates zero concentrations of carcinogens in foods. It is obviously a paradoxical law that insists that zero concentrations exist when science tells us they do not.

Testing

Over the years, regulatory agencies have developed a series of tests to determine whether a given substance has adverse effects. Most tests used the "brute force" approach: Animals were fed maximum amounts of the substance in question. Often it was not clear whether the observed effect was a result of the large amount of test substance added to the diet or to a toxic effect that could be extrapolated to normal levels of usage. By 1973, however, new techniques had given the Food and Drug Administration (FDA) confidence in its ability to distinguish between important and unimportant effects in toxicology and specifically in carcinogenesis.

The FDA has a variety of effective tests, but in some areas, we still do not know enough to ask the right questions. One of the reasons that research and knowledge are lagging in these areas of potential hazard is the almost single-minded concern with cancer. This concern in relation to the food supply has focused mostly on food additives and environmental contaminants. I must, however, raise this question: Do foodborne carcinogens deserve the attention and funding dollars that they now receive? In 1981 a special committee of the National Academy of Sciences reported that about 30% of the cancer hazard in the United States was associated with smoking, 35% with dietary patterns, 2% with contamination of the food supply, and less than 1% with food additives. The committee emphasized that the simplest action that the American public could take to produce the most immediate decline in the cancer rate was to ban the use of tobacco. The bulk of public health research dollars, however, has gone to the issues of food contamination and food additives. Despite these facts, regulatory agencies must respond to the demands of the public as expressed by Congress, and food contaminants and additives are currently at the top of the list.

Risk Assessment

It was not until the 1970s and the advent of risk-assessment techniques that the FDA was able to make rational decisions regarding the relative risk of various substances. For the first time a regulatory policy stated explicity that because everything had a risk, risks could be compared, decisions made, and the maximum risk reduced. The risk assessment policy also allowed the regulator to emphasize that safety is not absolute, but rather a point on a continuum that begins in an area called "unsafe" and ends in another area called "safe." The point at which the transition from safe to unsafe is established depends on the society's need and desires regarding a standard. It is important to remember that risk assessments are complicated.

Because there is still much we do not understand about the underlying mechanisms in these biological processes, the assessment is fundamentally a statistical model applied to a series of biological events. Accepting the results of a model often requires a leap of faith: Does the response of a given number of animals represent the response of the universe of animals? The response, therefore, must also be confirmed as biologically consistent and reasonable.

In a discussion of risk assessment, many people like to discuss risk-benefit evaluations. I do not believe that it is possible to do a risk-benefit calculation when it comes to foods. To whom does the benefit side of the equation apply? Does the development of a new food additive benefit the producer or the public? Further, in what units should the benefit be expressed: dollars? Increasing shelf life? Risk will always be expressed in terms of human life or health, and it is difficult to convert benefit to those units. The use of the dollar as the unit of benefit is not acceptable to the American public. For foods in particular and health in general, the most rational approach asks not about benefit but about risk: What are the risks of using a new substance compared to the risks of not using it?

Microbiology

Chemophobia is an interesting phenomenon in contemporary American society. Although Americans fear chemical food additives, there is a consensus among food-safety experts that the major problems of human health are associated with microbiological, not chemical, contamination of the food supply. For example, between 20 and 80 million cases of foodborne disease occur annually in the United States. This is a disease entity that has been largely ignored by the American health professions; most cases are not life-threatening and, until recently, most enteric disease was attributed to unknown causes. Today, advances in biological techniques have identified foodborne microorganisms as the cause of much of this disease. Much greater gains in public health could be made by giving more attention to sanitation and the control of these microorganisms than by increasing control of chemical hazards. This is not to say that chemical hazards should not be monitored and controlled, but rather that resources must be shared with more important and immediate issues such as food sanitation.

Diet and Nutrition

Dietary guidelines have become a way of life for governments in all parts of the world. They are not only a major component of health education but also major marketing tools. Not surprisingly, there is great commercial interest in the development of foods for dietary purposes. Unfortunately, too much energy is directed toward the "selling" of nutrition information rather than toward developing a substantial data base to reduce controversy in this area of nutrition.

When discussing the safety of diet, we generally concentrate on nutritional balances, excesses, and deficiencies. Determination of nutrient requirements under laboratory conditions, however, does not necessarily establish the real requirement in the real world. We should determine appropriate models and use them to evaluate true nutrient requirements rather than using the current approach to determining the Recommended Daily Allowances (RDAs).

The RDAs originally were designed to compare *population* nutrient intakes for the estimation of nutrient needs. They were never intended to be used to evaluate *individual* nutrient requirements. As a result, conservative assumptions are built into the RDAs to assure that 99% of the population receives its dietary needs. It is a necessary corollary that the RDAs will exceed the nutrient requirements by one or more orders of magnitude for a substantial segment of the population. Because recent research in nutrition indicates that nutrient excess can be as harmful as nutrient deficiency, a new approach to the estimation of human nutrient requirements must be developed. Unfortunately, neither government agencies nor private institutions are investing much money in this mundane but absolutely vital area of human health research.

Finally, what are our concerns about the future of the food supply and its origins? Together, traditional agricultural research and food science and technology have successfully met the goals of national policies designed to alleviate hunger and nutritional deficiency. In the process, however, new questions have been raised about agricultural policy. For example, the recognition of the role of diet in biological processes has led to an increasing awareness of the need for proper nutrition to prevent disease and enable a satisfactory lifestyle. More specifically, the results of research in chronic disease and public health indicate that we must formulate a food and agricultural research policy that incorporates considerations of good health. Consequently, nutrition and toxicology must become major elements in our planning for agriculture and the food industry for the rest of the century. We need explicit national and international food policies based on improving not only the quantity of food but also the quality. The acknowledgment that productivity alone cannot be the goal of agricultural policy in industrialized nations will be an important policy shift. It will place additional pressure on the scientific community to produce new strains of animals and plants to meet these health needs and on the food industry to produce new products that better meet our developing understanding of the requirements for maintenance and improvement of health.

We must also consider the changing nature of food itself. It is now possible to modify traditional foods to develop new food sources. An enormous inventory of new techniques includes plant cell and protoplast culture, plant regeneration, somatic hybridization, embryo transfer, and recombinant DNA techniques.

These exciting innovations may, however, have health or safety problems that must be assessed. I have identified five categories of these new food products, each with its unique health-related problems:

- New constructions or processing of traditional foods, e.g., irradiation
- Nontraditional foods for which some human experience exists, e.g., foods derived from yeast
- Products constructed from nontraditional raw materials such as certain fungi
- Products of chemical synthesis promoted for their functional or organoleptic properties
- Products constructed from or consisting solely of organisms that result from genetic manipulations

Each of these new product categories represents a unique and formidable challenge to those charged with assuring the safety and nutritional value of the food supply. Developing better ways to evaluate the safety of novel foods is a scientific challenge that regulators must face as the food industry uses science and technology to develop new food choices. Traditional approaches to evalute safety by examining the effects of exaggerated doses will not work for new food products.

Superimposed on all these issues remains the problem of public acceptance and recognition of the need for these new products. The need for public education will continue to be great. Public perceptions to a large extent drive the efforts of regulatory agencies. One must never forget that the public elects Congress and that Congress controls the budgets of these agencies and decides where their regulatory efforts will be directed.

The only way to ensure the level of food safety required by modern society is to develop cooperation between innovator and regulator. Regulatory agencies must have the support of both science and industry. If the regulator is to be rational, it must know the most recent scientific research and also must be kept abreast of the recent advances in industry. When a regulatory agency is uninformed, it can only respond negatively to petitions for approval of new food substances. Without cooperation, the continuing conflict between the separate agendas of industry and public-interest groups will result in the loss of important new technologies that might improve the well-being of people throughout the world.

Suggested Reading

Miller SA. Toxicology and food safety regulations. Arch Toxicol 1987; 60:212-6.

Miller SA. Scientific decision making from a national policy perspective. Food Drug Cosmetic Law, in press.

Miller SA, Taylor M. Historical development of food regulation. In: Middlekauff R, Shubik P, eds. International Handbook of Food Regulation. Marcel Dekker, New York:1989.

Skinner K, Miller SA. Food safety regulation. In: Clayson DB, Krewski D, Munro I, eds. Toxicological Risk Assessment, Vol. 2. Boca Raton, FL: CRC Press, 1985:109-18.

8

Future Directions in Food Technology

MARCUS KAREL, Ph.D.*

Driving Forces and Resistance in Food Technological Innovations

Innovations in food technology depend on several interacting factors: 1) the real or the perceived needs and wants of the consumer, 2) legal and other regulatory issues, 3) the presence of adequate consumer education, 4) economic issues, and 5) scientific and engineering advances. I will review the effects these factors will have on our ability to change and improve the ways in which we produce, preserve, and distribute foods. I will discuss the last category, scientific and engineering advances, in greatest detail.

*Massachusetts Institute of Technology, Cambridge, Massachusetts, and Rutgers University, New Brunswick, New Jersey.

The Consumer

The attitudes of the consuming public are probably the most important factor in marketing food. In addition to taste, there are currently three major consumer concerns regarding food products: health and safety, convenience, and cost. Both the public and medical experts now recognize the importance of diet in the maintenance of good health and the promotion of longevity. The prescription of simple dietary guidelines for a long and healthy life, however, is made difficult by the complexity of the interactions between diet and health. The field is consequently wide open to the promoters of specific dietary measures, some meritorious and some of little value. The consumer is therefore extremely susceptible to diet fashions. Current dietary components prominently identified with good health by the public include calcium, fiber (especially from oats), and omega-3 fatty acids. Those currently identified with ill health include pesticide residues, coconut and palm oils, and cholesterol. Although some of these concerns are transitory, the trend toward associating specific food components with health and well-being is likely to persist. Caloric content, cholesterol, and carcinogens will remain key concerns.

Consumers are also concerned with the convenience of a food or food product. Changes in lifestyles have generated a demand for "fast foods," snacks (including those with a controlled nutrient content), foods easily prepared in a microwave oven, and prepared, portion-controlled foods. The desire for convenience, however, is paired with increased attention to perceived quality. The perception of quality is, of course, subjective, but I believe that the appearance of "gourmet" prepared foods and the widespread acceptance of "ethnic" foods have resulted in improved standards of quality for convenience foods.

The consumer is also concerned about the cost of foods. In spite of the unprecedented economic growth of the past several years, the discretionary income of most consumers has not increased.

Legal and Regulatory Issues

The marketing of food is regulated by a myriad of complex laws and regulations, administered by several agencies within several government departments. As a result, the regulatory review process for the development of new food products or processes is costly and often long. It is not unusual to see lags of decades between the perfection of a process or ingredient and the regulatory approval for its use in commercial food production.

Consumer Education

Responsible education is the desirable solution to the confusion that exists among consumers regarding the various claims linking diet and health. Unfortunately, most consumer education regarding diet and health is promulgated through radio, newspapers, magazines, and television, and the inherent commerical characteristics of those organizations often interfere with the straightforward reporting of information about issues of diet and health. Emphasis is often given to the sensational or dramatic aspects of such as issue.

Advertising is another powerful medium in both the education and, unfortunately, the miseducation of the consumer. Both the food industry and consumer groups have often oversimplified or, on occasion, misrepresented scientific evidence in advertisements in support of their various points of view.

The complexity of the issues and the public airing of various conflicts within the scientific community have made the public skeptical of established views. Paradoxically, however, the skepticism is combined with a naive acceptance of unconventional views about diet and health. The public disillusionment with "authoritative" pronouncements from an established source, be it government, university, church, or professional society, makes public education in science a difficult and often thankless task. It is, however, the responsibility of the food scientist to continue to present the facts, without oversimplification and despite the occasional public mistrust.

Economic Issues

The development of new food products and processes in the food industry is driven by the profit motive. Inducements to innovation include not only the improved ability to convince a consumer to purchase a product, but also the producer's need to reduce costs.

The most prominent feature of the present industrial economy is its globality. Raw materials can now be obtained from all over the world. The food industry has been able to overcome some labor-cost increases by importing labor for agricultural tasks or raw food materials from faraway places. The global nature of food processing has greatly increased the requirements for quality control of imported foodstuffs. Real dangers of the transfer of microbial pathogens or other contaminants require constant vigilance of the quality-control systems.

Another characteristic of the food industry is the accelerating trend toward automation and computer control of production, storage, and distribution of foods.

Scientific and Engineering Advances

Economic incentives alone are inadequate to produce technical innovations. New scientific discoveries must also occur. In many cases, in fact, scientific advances generate the development of incentives.

In the coming years the food industry is likely to be revolutionized by advances that have been made in three fields of inquiry: computer science, genetic engineering, and materials science. The availability of new computer software and hardware has already had an enormous impact on practices in the food and related industries. One of the most visible impacts of new computing products has been in analytical and industrial instrumentation. Modern analytical methodologies depend on computers, and software is now available that performs a range of tasks from the simulation of molecular motion to the collection, calculation, and recording of analytical data. Process control and automated manufacturing is also dependent on modern high-speed computers.

Other functions of the food industry that have been influenced by computers include inventory maintenance and the control of storage, distribution, and merchandising. We are now familiar with bar codes and scanners, which enable checkout-counter personnel to record and display the price and other encoded information about each item of merchandise. "First-in, first-out" inventory management is now possible, and systems are on the horizon that will combine integration of effects of time and temperature. Such systems will enable inventory management on the basis of "most-aged, first-out."

Advances in genetic engineering have also begun to affect the food industry. We now can transfer the ability to produce a given enzyme from higher organisms to microorganisms. For example, an enzyme heretofore resident only in cows at a certain age can be transferred to an organism that can be grown in a vat under controlled conditions, and the enzyme may be produced and isolated in large quantities for use in food processing. Genetic engineering is also being used to speed breeding in animals.

Food materials science is the study of the relations between the structure and composition of food and its functional properties. It provides the foundation for the development of engineered foods. The importance of advances in this field need hardly be stressed in the age of "reformed" meats, surimi, diet drinks with alternative sweeteners, and the development of fat substitutes. Traditional food-production methods relied on the selection of existing plant or animal products which, by chance, had certain desired qualities. The concept underlying engineered food is the delivery of the desired characteristic (for example, sweetness, a fat-like mouthfeel, or a particular texture, color, or appearance) through the selection of ingredients appropriate for that characteristic, based on their chemical composition or their physical structure.

Advances in computer science, genetic engineering, or materials science, however, do not guarantee progress in the food industry. The industry must provide bridges for the transfer of technologies and the adaptation of the technologies to the specific needs of the industry and of consumers. Unfortunately, the current progress in bridge-building is not entirely satisfactory. I believe the food industry must urgently undertake the following steps:

1. Develop a major effort to relate the function of ingredients in food products to their physicochemical properties, molecular structure, and biological activity.
2. Specify requirements for "engineered" ingredients in molecular terms.

3. Resolve the controversy about natural versus "nature-identical" sources.
4. Adopt a long-term view in research and development.
5. Develop an understanding of the processes (biosynthesis, biodegradation, and chemical reactions) at work in the generation of key ingredients (for example, flavors).

For a number of reasons, many major food companies in the United States have been forced to concentrate on relatively short-term financial goals. As a result, basic research efforts in the materials science of foods have been reduced or postponed.

Computer and materials science technology have yet to give us a vital element for the reproducible, quality-conscious production of foods: the ability to measure a particular quality characteristic during the production process. The future will probably revolve around such a capability, which will allow us to adjust the severity of the process to the demands of the raw material.

Basic research in food biotechnology in the United States is going on in small, venture-capital-funded companies. The major efforts in this field, however, are underway in Europe and Japan.

Specific Technological Developments

Supercritical Fluid Extraction

Supercritical fluid applications have received much attention in recent years. Much attention has been devoted to the potential for this process in the removal of cholesterol from butter and eggs. The future of this particular application is uncertain, however, because of its high cost. I estimate that the reduction of the cholesterol content in butter by a factor of 10 would cost $2 to $3 per pound of butter, surely a prohibitive cost. The extraction of expensive volatile flavors, however, or the removal of more soluble compounds from expensive raw materials (for example, caffeine from coffee) seems more promising.

Food Irradiation

Ionizing radiation is effective in the: 1) destruction or sterilization of insects, 2) prevention of sprouting by tubers, 3) softening of cellulose-containing plant materials, and 4) pasteurization or sterilization of foods. The current status of irradiation as a food-processing application, however, is extremely uncertain because of public mistrust of any processes connected to nuclear energy. Of course, the radiation applied to foods does not transfer to people who eat the food. Concerns about the safety of this process are its potential to produce undesirable chemical compounds and its effect on workers in food factories with radioisotope installations. Irradiation is also capable of producing off-flavor in some food materials.

I believe the following applications for irradiation are the most cost-effective and safe:

1. Destruction of insects in fruits and vegetables shipped across state and national boundaries and in grain shipped across national boundaries
2. Pasteurization of poultry, fish, and feedstuffs to eliminate such disease-causing organisms as *Salmonella, Yersinia,* and *Campylobacter*
3. Sterilization of spices, which may carry disease-causing organisms
4. Elimination of sprouting in some plant species

At present, legal restriction on the irradiation of foodstuffs is severe, and application is limited to grain disinfestation (USSR), pasteurization (Europe), and inhibition of potato sprouting (Japan). Petitions are currently pending for permission to irradiate poultry to eliminate *Salmonella, Yersinia*, and *Campylobacter*. If the public concern can be overcome, irradiation is likely to be used in combination with other food-processing methods for spice sterilization, insect eradication, pathogen elimination, and, in combination with refrigeration, extension of poultry and seafood shelf life. It might also be used in the sterilization of containers for aseptic packaging.

Electromagnetic Radiation

Our innate desire to overcome the limitations imposed on us by nature is strong, and it has been instrumental in effecting vast technological change. Unfortunately, this desire can also lead us on wild goose chases. Many allegedly miraculous food-preservation methods have been developed, including laser processing and high-magnetic fields. The true physical principles of food preservation, however, remain limited. To destroy microorganisms, thermal, ionizing, or mechanical energy must be applied, or the organisms must be physically removed from the food and separated from the edible food constituents. The latter possibility is one of the applications for membrane processing.

Membrane Processes

Membrane processes are common now, but new combinations have the potential to produce novel products. All membrane processes use the membrane pores for separation. Components are driven through the pores by pressure (reverse osmosis), an electric charge (electrodialysis), a difference in concentrations (dialysis), or a combination of these forces. New applications, for example, may deacidify food liquids by electrodialysis, then concentrate the deacidified product by reverse osmosis.

Engineered Foods

Engineered foods have been modified or assembled to achieve key performance characteristics. For instance, a can of diet soda which contains aspartame has two such characteristics: sweetness and reduced caloric content. A major advantage for the makers of engineered foods is the flexibility of such foods. For example, in making bread, candy bars, or snack foods, one may use wheat, rye, or corn flour, and vary the sweetener or the fat source. This flexibility is important in the face of variations in the market for raw foodstuffs. In an engineered food, coconut oil could be replaced with other fats, or corn could be replaced with another grain if, for example, a corn-producing region had been contaminated by aflatoxin. Substitutions in the raw materials of engineered foods may also be made in response to fluctuations in price, or changes in political conditions or consumer attitudes. For example, the ability to engineer foods has enabled food manufacturers to take advantage of the recent popularity of oat bran by adding it to a variety of foods.

Engineered foods also offer flexibility in obtaining a desired characteristic. For example, the process for making hard cookies can be transformed into one for soft-center cookies by replacing part of the crisp, crystallizable component, sucrose, with a center that has a different sugar or starch, which inhibits crystallization. The crisp center then becomes a soft center. In low-calorie foods, one could engineer the perception of fat and generate a market for fat substitutes. Other desired characteristics in engineered foods might include the method of preparation in the home. Suitability for microwave cooking, for example, has been engineered into many products.

It should be noted that an engineered product may use no synthetic components. Bread is an engineered product. It has built into it a certain number of air cells, a crust, a crumb (the mix of flavor compounds produced by yeast), and a caloric content. Engineering used in the context of food processing simply means the use of specific components to achieve desired characteristics.

A primary limitation on the production of new engineered foods is the desire of the food industry to maintain the "natural" image for the purposes of labeling and advertising. For example, benzaldehyde synthesized from toluene is a fraction of the cost of benzaldehyde derived from almond oil, but the less expensive, chemically identical benzaldehyde cannot be called "natural." A success story in this controversy is the development, use, and successful marketing of aspartame, which has fulfilled an important need in calorie-controlled foods. It took a long time for aspartame to be accepted, but it is now a major component of engineered drinks and many other foods.

Other areas in which considerable potential exists are polymer and lipid engineering. Polymers might be engineered to carry attached functional groups that can signal the presence of *Salmonella* in a product or to impart a specific taste, flavor, or appearance. Lipid engineering could be used to control caloric or other characteristics. There is currently considerable pressure to develop fat substitutes. Unfortunately, some noncaloric lipids have serious problems: Those that are absorbed even slightly must be studied at length for their effect on the liver and other organs, and those that are not absorbed may present gastrointestinal problems, including diarrhea or anal leakage. Polymer engineering, as in the use of microparticulated protein, may therefore represent a more successful approach to the development of a fat substitute.

Flavor engineering is another area with enormous potential for the food industry. We have not yet duplicated the flavors that exist in nature, but this ability will come. We already have almost limitless analytical capabilities. Now we need more knowledge about the effects on our brain of given molecules or compounds. We need to know how these substances interact with the sensors in our nose and mouth and how that signal is translated. When we have that information, we will see a revolution in flavor engineering as far-reaching as the revolution in genetic engineering.

The concept of engineering foods will become increasingly important in tailoring foods for groups with special food needs. Such groups include people who are dieting, have food-drug interaction problems, are at risk for atherosclerosis, and have allergies, and those in specific age groups. We will be able to tailor foods for specific health problems, whether they be inborn errors of metabolism or drug-induced illness. We also will produce sterile foods for patients undergoing chemotherapy, whose immune systems are temporarily unable to protect them. Such foods may also support therapy for people with AIDS. Foods designed to reduce the risk of atherosclerosis will be produced, because this disease is the major limiting factor in the average life span, and because many of the decision-makers who determine the fate of research dollars are at high risk for atherosclerosis and coronary heart disease.

The brain will be the site of the next scientific revolution, and the discoveries in this area of research will enable great advances in food and flavor engineering. I believe we will know 1) how to control the appetite, 2) where the sensory input pathways are located, 3) how to control satiety, and 4) why the same level of a given amino acid may affect one person and not another.

Advances in Packaging

The same principle of tailoring being used in food composition is now being used, and will be used on a much higher scale, in the manufacture of food-packaging materials. We can tailor the atmosphere in a package to be compatible with the quality of its contents. This process will require appropriate sensors and the ability to control precisely for quality. Preservation of food by controlled-atmosphere packaging depends on rigorous quality control of the production system.

"Active packaging" will also come into use. Active packaging uses surfaces or accessible interiors of the packaging materials as reaction sites. One can produce packaging materials that will, for example, absorb oxygen, remove water, or absorb ethylene, so that the ripening of fresh fruits and vegetables is delayed. In addition to absorbing or removing undesirable atmospheric components, systems may be incorporated into packages that will release or generate flavors, inhibitors, antioxidants, or other active atmospheric components.

Another area in which we will make great advances is shelf-life prediction. A package can contain a system that will inform us not only that a given product has been on a shelf for n days, but that it has experienced, for example, temperature conditions that are equivalent to $(n + 20)$ or $(n + y)$ standard days. Under these circumstances, a decision can be made to accept or reject a product on the basis not only of age, but also age plus abuse. A manufacturer could direct the distribution of products such that he would first ship products that were likely to spoil sooner, based on age plus abuse, rather than shipping products based on their age alone. Food manufacturers could realize enormous savings by the consequent reduction of merchandise rejection by retailers.

Conclusion

The major characteristics of food-preservation techniques in the early 21st century will include flexibility, the combination of existing methods into a single new process, and computer-aided control. Flexibility will take the form of the interchangeability of raw materials; components will be substituted on the basis of function. Existing production methods, such as electron beams, heat exchangers, microwaves, or the control of water activity, gas composition, or the release of preservatives, will be synthesized into a single new process stringently controlled through a combination of sensors and computers. Computer-aided control will include real-time response, the monitoring of specific sensors for control of specific properties, and advanced data acquisition and retrieval systems. If there is an appropriate emphasis on basic research in these areas vital to the food industry, the potential for advances in food engineering, production, and packaging is tremendous.

Suggested Reading

Graham JC, Green LC, Roberts MJ. In search of safety: chemicals and cancer risk. Cambridge, MA: Harvard University Press, 1988.

Heylin M. Credibility. Chem Eng News 1989(May 22):3.

Hui YH. United States food laws, regulations, and standards. New York: Wiley-Interscience; 1979.

Labuza TP, Breene WM. Applications of "active packaging" for improvement of shelf-life and nutritional quality of fresh and extended shelf life foods. J Food Process Preserv 1989;13:1-69.

McHugh M, Krukonis V. Supercritical fluid extraction, principles and practice. Boston: Butterworth, 1986.

Seltzer R. Alar on apples. Chem Eng News 1989(May 22):4.

Wells JH, Singh RP. A quality based inventory issue policy for perishable foods. J Food Process Preserv 1989;12(4):271-92.

Whitney LF. What expert systems can do for the food industry. Food Technol 1989;43(5):120.

9

Dietary Fatty Acids and Cholesterol

WILLIAM E. CONNOR, M.D.*

Atherosclerosis and Coronary Heart Disease

Atherosclerosis afflicts well over half the population of the United States, and is a particularly lethal disease in men aged 40 to 60. We have to regard atherosclerosis as a disorder of fat or lipid metabolism, much as diabetes is regarded as a disorder of carbohydrate metabolism. Lesions in the coronary arteries of patients who have died from atherosclerosis have two components: a lipid portion and a blood clot or thrombus. The lipid portion has narrowed an artery in these patients, and the thrombus has closed it. The formation of both the lipid lesion and the thrombus are influenced by dietary factors.

*Oregon Health Sciences University, Portland, Oregon.

The development of coronary heart disease is a three-stage process. Stage one always involves abnormal levels of plasma lipids and lipoproteins; stage two is the formation of fatty lesions in the arteries, that is, atherosclerosis. In the third stage, a thrombus blocks a coronary artery, and the heart is damaged as a result of an insufficient blood supply.

Approximately 1% of the world's hypercholesterolemia, a high blood cholesterol level, is the consequence of heredity. In the other 99% of individuals with hypercholesterolemia, the condition develops because of lifestyle, particularly dietary habits. Other risk factors that contribute to the development of coronary heart disease include hypertension, that is, high blood pressure, cigarette smoking, stress, and physical inactivity. To reduce the prevalence of coronary heart disease, we must reduce the current high levels of blood cholesterol in our population.

We can determine an individual's risk for developing coronary heart disease by measuring serum cholesterol levels. We are born with a cholesterol level of 70 mg/dl, and, in human and other primate populations that have little coronary disease, the level throughout life is approximately 120 to 140 mg/dl. These levels would be safe goals over a lifetime, although the view has become commonplace that a safe everyday cholesterol level is below 180 mg/dl.

Cholesterol, Fats, and Lipoproteins

Cholesterol and triglycerides (fats) are insoluble in water, but are transported in the body in plasma, an aqueous medium. These fats, therefore, must be packaged and covered with a water-soluble protein envelope. They are transported in the form of lipoproteins, of which there are four different classes, and the proportions of each are affected by diet. The chylomicron, the first class of lipoproteins, results from the ingestion of dietary fat and cholesterol. It is formed in the lining of the intestines, enters the bloodstream, and after approximately 4 to 6 hours, it disappears. This particle is not atherogenic; i.e., it will not cause fatty degeneration of the arteries, because it is too large to get between the cells lining the artery and begin a deposit. A chylomicron is, however, acted on by an enzyme that breaks it into much smaller particles, and these particles can adhere to the arterial walls. The major point is that simply be eating fat, we produce a particle in the bloodstream that can cause atherosclerosis.

The second class of lipoproteins, very-low-density lipoprotein (VLDL), is synthesized by the liver. The liver is vital to both the production and the disposal of cholesterol and triglyceride. VLDL is secreted by the liver when we are not eating fats and other foods. It is released into the bloodstream and is responsible for triglyceride transport during a period of fasting. Like the chylomicron, the VLDL also gives rise to a remnant particle that does cause fatty degeneration of the arteries.

The third class of lipoproteins, low-density lipoprotein (LDL), is the most atherogenic. It is much smaller than the other lipoproteins and is the chief carrier of cholesterol. Over our lifetimes, LDL and its component, apolipoprotein B, deposit most of the cholesterol in our arterial walls. These deposits cause atherosclerosis and, later, coronary heart disease. The amounts of LDL also rise with age. As we grow older, our body's ability to regulate the amount of this particle diminishes.

High-density lipoproteins (HDL), the fourth class, help protect our arteries from high cholesterol levels. Whereas high levels of chylomicrons, VLDL, or LDL are harmful, a high HDL level is beneficial.

Dietary Intake and Coronary Heart Disease

Diet contributes to the development and, conversely, the prevention of coronary heart disease. The major dietary components affecting heart health are cholesterol and fat. Further consideration must also be given to the type of fat: saturated, polyunsaturated, or monounsaturated. It can now be firmly stated that cholesterol and saturated fat give rise to the development of coronary heart disease; and their presence raises the level of LDL in the blood. Polyunsaturated fat, however, tends to lower cholesterol and LDL levels, and some studies have shown that ingestion of liquid vegetable oils that contain omega-6 fatty acids (particularly linoleic acid) lowers cholesterol levels. Concern, however, that these fatty acids may promote cancer when ingested at high levels has kept them from being used in the American diet as a tool to lower serum cholesterol levels.

The omega-3 fatty acids, primarily derived from fish, do lower serum cholesterol and triglyceride levels, but are not likely to cause cancer. In fact, the reverse may be true, and these fats are now on the cutting edge of therapy for coronary heart disease.

The ingestion of excessive calories, particularly fat calories, stimulates overproduction of cholesterol and fat by the liver; therefore excessive caloric intake alone will cause increased blood levels of fat and cholesterol. Reducing the amount of fat that we consume has become very important. We often are advised to replace the fat in our diet with carbohydrate, but it is important to use the right type of carbohydrate. The simple carbohydrates, such as sugars, tend to elevate lipid levels, but the complex, starchy carbohydrates in beans, pasta, potatoes, rice, and bread do not. In fact, when the starchy carbohydrates are associated with fiber, particularly soluble fiber, there is a slight cholesterol-lowering effect. Some carbohydrate-containing foods, such as beans, contain a natural chemical substance called saponins. Saponins tend to interfere with cholesterol absorption and therefore may have a positive effect in the prevention of coronary heart disease.

When we substitute foods rich in complex carbohydrates for those rich in fats, we are not only replacing fat with carbohydrates to supply calories, we may also be replacing the fat with substances that help prevent cholesterol absorption or promote bile acid excretion. Foods that contain complex carbohydrates and fiber may therefore help prevent coronary heart disease through their interference with cholesterol metabolism.

The Liver and Cholesterol

The liver is the key organ in both the synthesis and removal of cholesterol. Liver cells have specific sites, called receptors, for removing

LDL and its accompanying cholesterol from the blood. An LDL receptor specifically recognizes an LDL molecule, removes the molecule from the bloodstream, and enables the liver cell to digest it. The liver cell digests everything in the LDL molecule *except* the cholesterol. The amount of cholesterol, therefore, builds up within the cell. Because too much cholesterol is harmful to a cell, each cell has a self-regulating mechanism designed to control the amount of intracellular cholesterol. If there is too much cholesterol in the cell, the self-regulating mechanism: 1) tells the cholesterol synthesis mechanism in the liver to reduce or stop its activity, 2) esterifies some of the cholesterol, and 3) reduces the number of LDL receptors on the liver cell. As these steps occur, the overload of cholesterol in the cell is reduced, and the cell is protected. As the number of LDL receptors is reduced, however, the level of LDL in the blood is raised.

If we eat cholesterol and saturated fat, therefore, we set this process in motion. The amount of cholesterol entering the liver cell increases and, to prevent excessive accumulation of intracellular cholesterol, the liver cell takes up less cholesterol from the blood. This in turn raises the level of LDL in the plasma.

Dietary Sources of Cholesterol and Fat

If we are to intervene successfully at a nutritional level to prevent excessive dietary intake of cholesterol, it is important to know the sources of cholesterol in the American diet. About 45% of the cholesterol we eat comes from egg yolk, and about half of that 45% is in processed foods in which the egg yolk is not visible. For example, cookies, doughnuts, pancake mixes, and similar foods have egg yolk that we don't know about and haven't chosen to eat. About 35% of our dietary cholesterol comes from meat, fish, and poultry, because all animal cells (and only animal cells) contain cholesterol. Most of that 35% comes from meat, because we eat more meat than fish or poultry. Dairy products provide 20%, but it should be noted that low-fat and fat-free dairy products, for example, skim milk or nonfat yogurt, contain virtually no cholesterol. Cholesterol in dairy products comes in the form of cheese, ice cream, whole milk, and butter. When designing a diet that will keep the LDL level in the blood as low as possible, these are important foods to consider.

The dietary sources of fat, particularly saturated fat, are also important. Only 6% of our fat intake comes from fruits, vegetables, grains, and beans, but the fats that these foods supply are largely omega-6 and omega-3 fatty acids, which are considered essential by many researchers. Forty-three percent of our fat intake comes from fats and oils, and half that amount is invisible because it is included in processed foods, e.g., cookies, doughnuts, etc. Technology in the food industry has developed these products in which the fat is invisible, and it should, therefore, be able to improve our overall health by modifying those fats. It should be possible, for example, to produce a vegetable oil almost devoid of saturated fat. Dairy products supply 11% of our fat, and meat, fish, poultry, and eggs supply the remaining 39%, most of that from fatty meat. If we want to lower the amount of fat in the American diet, we must decrease the consumption of these food products.

Saturated fats have varying effects on plasma cholesterol level. and this fact has created some confusion. Some saturated fats that are water-soluble do not elevate plasma cholesterol; others, particularly lauric, myristic, and palmitic fatty acids, do increase plasma cholesterol. The saturated fats that do elevate plasma cholesterol and LDL levels include coconut, palm, and palm kernel oils, butter fat, and beef, pork and lamb fats. Cocoa butter, the fat in chocolate, will also raise plasma cholesterol. Again, the consumption of foods or food products that contain cholesterol-raising saturated fats should be limited.

There are also food constituents that decrease plasma cholesterol. These include soluble fibers, provided by grains, fruits and legumes, and saponins, in a wide variety of foods, particularly alfalfa sprouts, beans, yams, and soybeans. Consumption of these foods in the American diet should be encouraged.

Omega-3 Fatty Acids and Coronary Heart Disease

Eskimos, whose diet is high in cholesterol and fat, do not have the expected amount of coronary heart disease. This fact has long been a mystery. The fat that they consume, however, is different from fats produced by land animals, because it contains omega-3 fatty acids. Omega-3, like omega-6 fatty acids, are probably essential fatty acids, in that they are required for certain biochemical functions but are not synthesized by our bodies. We can therefore obtain them only through diet.

An important effect of omega-3 fatty acids is believed to be the prevention of atherosclerosis and heart disease, and there is abundant epidemiological information to support the theory. Netherlanders who ate two or three meals of fish per week has less coronary disease compared with those who did not eat fish. The people of Japanese fishing villages ate twice the amount of fish and had half the amount of coronary heart disease as people in Japanese farming villages. Experimental data in pigs and monkeys have also shown that omega-3 fatty acids, in the form of cod liver oil or other fish oils, retarded the development of atherosclerosis.

Native Americans of the northwestern U.S. coast had a diet high in salmon before the coming of the white man—and a low incidence of coronary heart disease. In an effort to discover the mechanism by which omega-3 fatty acids reduce atherosclerosis, volunteers were fed one pound of fresh salmon per day for 28 days. It was discovered that omega-3 fatty acids from salmon change the membranes of the body, including those of red blood cells, platelets, liver cells, and perhaps even brain cells.

When an injury occurs to the lining of a blood vessel, platelets adhere to one another and to the injury, thereby forming a blood thrombus or clot. Such a clot is instrumental in coronary heart disease, because it can block a coronary blood vessel and stop blood supply to the heart. Omega-3 fatty acids change the membrane composition of platelets and make them less adherent, thereby making the formation of blood clots less likely. In addition, consumption of omega-3 fatty acids has generally been shown to reduce plasma concentrations of cholesterol and fat. The results from the salmon-diet study have been replicated in some instances by the use of fish oil in capsule form.

Goals for the Reduction of Coronary Heart Disease in the United States

The objectives of the U.S. Public Health Service for 1990 and beyond include reduction of the cholesterol level for adults 18 to 74 years old to 200 mg/dl or below. Our mean level is approximately 210 mg/dl, so there is a long way to go for many people. Children should have a level below 150 mg/dl. These are feasible objectives, but only if we change our lifestyle as a nation. If we do not reduce our cholesteral levels, atherosclerotic lesions can get worse. If, however, we can stop the progression of these lesions, we could avoid coronary heart disease. If cholesterol levels are lowered, these lesions can be stabilized and even improved. It is imperative, then, that we reduce our cholesterol levels.

Omega-3 Fatty Acids in the Growth and Development of Infants

There are two major sources for omega-3 fatty acids. The leaves and some nuts and seeds of plants produce α-linolenic acid, and plants of the oceans, rivers, and lakes (i.e., phytoplankton) produce the highly polyunsaturated forms EPA and DHA. The plankton are consumed by fish and shellfish, and when we eat these seafoods, we ingest omega-3 fatty acids that have been developed at the base of the aquatic food chain.

We begin life, by nature, with a diet of human milk, which has certain specficic constituents. Protein, interestingly, makes up only 6% of the total calories; carbohydrate, 36% (largely as lactose); and fat, a surprising 54% of the total calories in human milk. In comparison, most American adults eat approximately 40% of their total calories in fat, whereas most peoples of the world eat as little as 12% of their total calories from fat. Of the fat in human milk, 42% is saturated, 39% unsaturated, and 17.8% polyunsaturated. In addition, there is a large amount of cholesterol, approximately 50 mg/cup, so this is basically an atherogenic diet. However, it does not produce atherosclerosis in humans, because we consume it only during the short period of infancy when we need a high-fat diet for healthy growth and development.

The quality of the polyunsaturated fat in human milk is very important, a fact that has not been universally recognized in the preparation of artificial infant formulas. Human milk contains about 1.3% of its total fatty acids as omega-3 fatty acids. A good portion of that 1.3% is the aforementioned highly polyunsaturated DHA. Infant formulas that contain MCT oil (a synthetic oil) and corn oil as their sources of fat, however, have very little omega-3 fatty acid. In fact, the results of one study show that such formulas do not contain enough omega-3 fatty acids to produce proper development of the brain and retina. Infant formulas that use corn oil alone have a little more DHA, and those that use soy oil begin to approach the DHA levels of human milk. None of these formulas, however, matches the DHA concentration in human milk, and none contains preformed DHA, which is rich in the brain and retina. It is possible that the addition of DHA to these formulas would improve the development of the brain and retina in infants who consumed them.

An experiment to determine the effects of omega-3 fatty acid deficiency on the development of infants was performed in rhesus monkeys. Two different diets were fed: One contained soy oil and the other, safflower oil, which is deficient in omega-3 fatty acids. Typically, growth is used as a measure of development, and if a diet is inadequate, it will not produce good growth. Although appropriate growth occurred in the monkeys whose diet was deficient in omega-3 fatty acids, something else happened; at 4 weeks of age, they did not see as well as the monkeys in the control group. The monkeys whose diet was deficient had a vision of 20/90, and monkeys in the control group had a vision of 20/45; the lack of omega-3 fatty acids in the diet of infant monkeys impaired their vision by about half. In addition, retinal response to light was impaired in the deficient group.

We have long considered growth the most important characteristic of adequate nutrition. It is obvious, however, that when growth is normal but the development of vision is abnormal, then the development of such functions must be considered along with growth in the determination of adequate nutrition. Omega-3 deficiency results in normal growth, but reduced learning and abnormal vision; omega-6 deficiency produces growth retardation, skin lesions, reproductive failure, and a fatty liver. Each of these fatty acids, then, supplies something necessary for proper growth and development, and each must therefore be considered an individual essential fatty acid.

The recommended intakes of these two fatty acids for infants, based on studies of monkeys, are 6 to 8% of total calories from omega-6 and about 1% of total calories from omega-3 in the form of α-linolenic acid. Although the omega-3 content of human milk is adequate, most infant formulas have far too little.

The critical periods of life for omega-3 and omega-6 fatty acid intake include infancy and pregnancy, but we also need to develop a reserve of omega-3 fatty acids in the adipose tissue so they will be available for the body during an emergency when food intake may be diminished. Therefore, intake of both these fatty acids should continue throughout life, in amounts of at least 1% to 2% of total calories.

In summary, there is strong evidence that 1) the development of atherosclerosis depends on the foods that populations and individuals habitually consume and 2) the body needs a certain amount of essential fatty acids. As adults, we have the option to modify our diets to prevent the development of atherosclerosis and coronary heart disease. We also have the imperative to make certain that infants receive a diet that contains appropriate amounts of fatty acids to ensure their growth and development.

Suggested Reading

Connor SL, Connor WE. The New American Diet. New York; Simon & Schuster, 1986:410.

Connor WE, Connor SL. Dietary treatment of familial hypercholesterolemia. Arteriosclerosis 1989;9(Suppl I):91-105.

Connor WE, Connor SL. Diet, atherosclerosis and fish oil. In Stollerman H, Siperstein MD, eds. Advances in Internal Medicine, Vol. 35. Chicago, Year Book Publishers, 1989:139-72.

Connor WE, Neuringer M. Importance of dietary omega-3 fatty acids in retinal function and brain chemistry. In: Nutritional Modulation of Neural Function. San Diego, CA: Academic Press, 1988:191-201.

Harris WS. Fish oils and plasma lipid and lipoprotein metabolism in humans: a critical review. J Lipid Res 1989;30:785-807.

Neuringer M, Anderson GJ, Connor WE. The essentiality of n-3 fatty acids for the development and function of the retina and brain. Ann Rev Nutr 1988;8:517-41.

Neuringer M, Connor WE, Lin DS, Barstad L, Luck S. Biochemical and functional effects of prenatal and postnatal omega-3 fatty acids deficiency on retinal and brain in rhesus monkeys. Proc Natl Acad Sci USA 1986;83:4021-5.

10

Sugar

NORMAN KRETCHMER, M.D., Ph.D.*

History

The word sugar is used in our vocabulary in many forms, each of which has as its primary meaning "sweet." Recently, sugar has become an emotional issue for some consumers, based on the false assumption that anything that tastes so good cannot be good for you. In reality, years of research have shown that moderate sugar consumption poses no risk to health in most people. There are, however, a few exceptions in which sugar intake must be controlled for health reasons.

Agricultural domestication of plants apparently was initiated in the Neolithic period about 10,000 years ago. Figure 1 shows the areas in which various foods were first grown. The countries of the Andes, Peru, Bolivia, and Ecuador, were major sites in the development of agriculture. Potatoes and tomatoes originated in this area. Guatemala and El Salvador were the countries in which corn,

*University of California at Berkeley and Koret Center for Human Nutrition, San Francisco General Hospital, San Francisco, California.

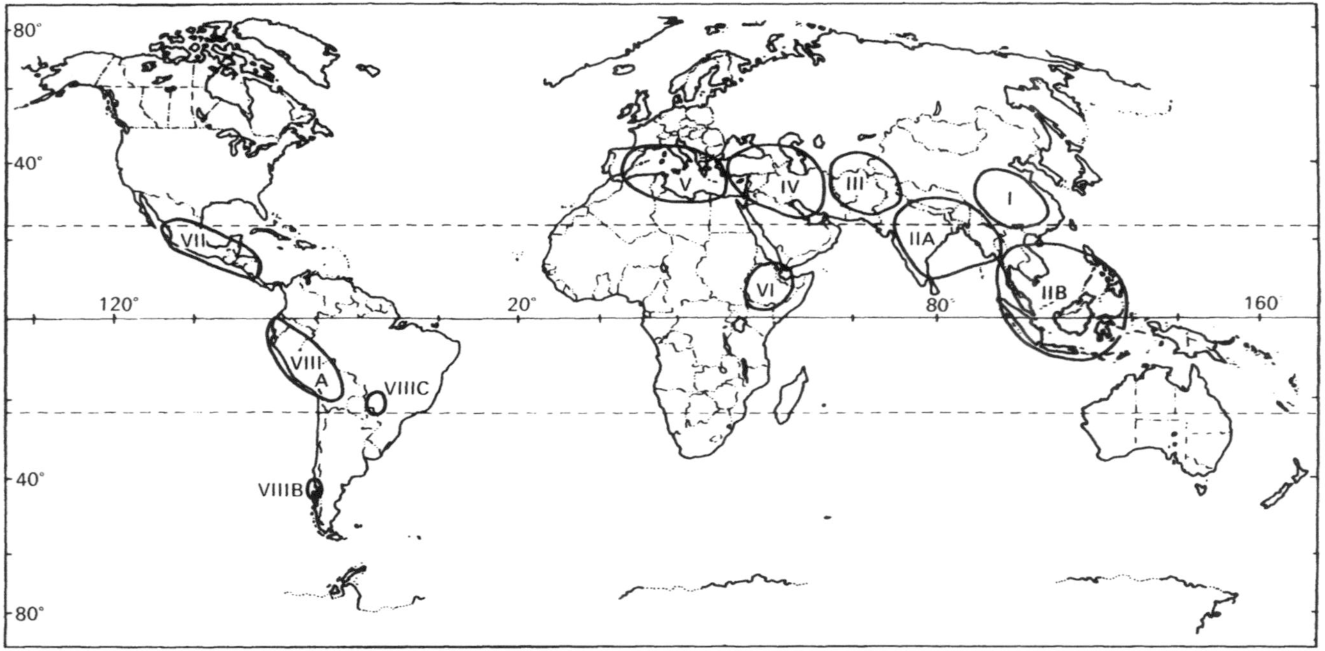

Figure 1 Centers of origin of cultivated plants. (After Vavilov NV, The Origin, Variation, Immunity and Breeding of Cultivated Plants. Translated by K. Starr Chester. New York: The Ronald Press, 1951.)

beans and squash originated. Yucca (manioc), now the major staple of West Africa, originated in South America (Brazil). From the lands around the Mediterranean came the olive. Wheat and farm animals originated in Asia Minor, a major agricultural hearth. Ethiopia gave birth to coffee and tef, a type of millet. Rice was first developed in China. Substances other than cane sugar were used as sweeteners; for example, during their exodus from Egypt, the Jews used manna, a glucose derivative excreted by insects. We generally think of sugar or sucrose as a derivative of sugar cane, but much of the sucrose used today is derived from the sugar beet.

Sugar cane as a crop originated in Papua-New Guinea about 8000 to 9000 years ago. During the ensuing thousands of years, it gradually moved west. Sugar arrived in the Western Hemisphere, primarily the Caribbean, shortly after the arrival of Columbus.

In 500 B.C., cane was brought to India and grown in the Ganges area. The Indians developed an industrial process to refine sugar cane to molasses. Sugar cultivation moved at the same time to southern China, then back to India, and during this time the first pure white crystalline product was produced. It then took more than 1000 years for sugar to move from China to Persia. In 640 A.D. the Chinese emperor sent a mission to India to study the techniques for extracting and purifying sugar so the Chinese could also produce the crystalline form of the sweetener. It is surprising that the contemporary Chinese diet contains almost no sugar. In 800 A.D. Buddhist monks took sugar to Japan. At approximately the same time, sugar moved from Persia to the Arabian peninsula, and the Arabs began to grow sugar on the islands of the Mediterranean. This activity influenced Egypt to become a producer of cane.

The Venetians were the major industrialists and marketers of the world during the Middle Ages. They sent products all over the world, and Venice became a major sugar-refining center around 1000 A.D. Sugar was still unknown in northern Europe and probably was brought into the European diet as a result of the Crusades. When the Crusaders arrived in Jerusalem, they saw sugar cane growing on the islands and the coast. They, of course, enjoyed the taste of sugar. Some Crusaders grew sugar while they were in the Middle

East; they took it back to Europe in 1200 A.D. It is believed that sugar was available at first only to the nobles in the court of Charlemagne. Sometime later, Marco Polo was impressed by the production of sugar he had seen during his travels to and from China and brought it with him to southern Europe.

Sugar was introduced into the Canary Islands during the 15th century, and in 1492 Columbus took sugar cane from the Canaries to the Caribbean. The physical environment of the Caribbean islands was conducive to the growth of sugar. There was a vociferous demand for sugar, primarily from England and France, and the sugar trade spread rapidly.

The slave trade between Africa and the Caribbean originated from the need for labor for the cane fields of the Caribbean islands. The so-called triangular route was begun: Europe to Africa to the Caribbean and back to Europe. The cultivation of sugar cane was introduced in Brazil and the Caribbean by Portuguese slave traders who also took their slaves from Africa. Sugar plantations operated by slave labor became the prominent feature of the Caribbean islands and parts of neighboring North and South America. Sugar from the Caribbean was first introduced into Europe in 1561 in the Spanish markets, and soon factories for refining sugar were being built throughout Europe.

The British entered the sugar industry and established sugar plantations in Barbados, Jamaica, and other Caribbean islands. The French also had established sugar plantations in the Caribbean on Martinique, Guadeloupe, and other islands, but with the advent of the Napoleonic wars and the British blockade, the French were cut off from Caribbean sugar. Napoleon was concerned about the loss of sugar, and sent engineers to Germany to learn the technique, developed by Margraff, to manufacture sugar from the white beet. Napoleon built beet-sugar plants in France, but they were never put into full production.

Before 1865, the Caribbean had approximately 80% of all the slaves in the world. By 1865, slavery was illegal in the United States, and the major production of sugar moved from the southern United States to Cuba. Cultivation of the plant spread to Central America, primarily the coastal regions. Sugar plantations began to develop with a west-east diffusion, and they now encircle the globe. Today, the major sugar producers in the world include not only Brazil, Hawaii, and the countries of the Caribbean, but also Australia, the Pacific islands, Indonesia, and much of Polynesia. Most of the sugar from beets is produced in the United States and the USSR.

In 1900, approximately 8 metric tons of sugar were produced; by 1981, sugar production was in the many millions of tons. The only groups whose diets did not include sugar were Eskimos and some hunter-gatherer societies. Today even these groups have readily taken sugar into their diets.

The United States government subsidizes sugar to maintain a specific price level. Sugar production increased steadily until the 1970s, after which sales of domestic and imported sugars declined considerably. Corn-syrup sweeteners have decreased the market for sugar. Almost all non-diet soft drinks in the United States now contain corn-syrup sweeteners. Although per-capita sugar consumption has declined (its zenith in the United States was approximately 100 lb per capita; it has now fallen to approximately 61 lb), the use of corn sweeteners has almost tripled, and the per-capita consumption of all sweeteners has remained at about 125 lb.

Physiology

Sucrose is the common table sugar. All common sugars contain glucose, the primary carbohydrate used by mammals for energy. Some sugars contain fructose (e.g., those in honey or corn syrup) or galactose (e.g., those in milk or connective tissue). Fructose, as honey, has been a major sweetener in the diet of the Middle East for many years. Maltose (glucose and glucose) is the final product of starch. Lactose (glucose and galactose) is present in the milks of all mammals except seals, sea lions, and walruses of the Pacific basin.

Fructose crosses the intestinal membrane by facilitative diffusion. Glucose requires energy and a carrier to be transported across the intestinal membrane. Glucose and fructose, the components of sucrose, can enter the bloodstream only if sucrose has been digested in the small intestine. The digestion of sucrose requires the enzyme sucrase, which is present only in the brush-border membrane of epithelial cells that line the small intestine. If the amount of sucrase is deficient, the ability to digest sucrose is impaired. The undigested sucrose molecule will pass intact into the large intestine, which in turn causes water to pass into the large intestine through osmotic action. Colonic bacteria ferment the sucrose into carbon dioxide, hydrogen, methane, and fatty acids, such as acetic acid and propionic acid. The fermentation results in flatulence and eventually fermentative diarrhea. Excess undigested sucrose will move passively across the intestinal membrane into the bloodstream, and it will be excreted intact by the kidney. If sucrase is present in the intestine in sufficient amounts, however, the disaccharide sucrose is readily digested into the monosaccharides fructose and glucose.

Some animals do not like sugar; others love it. Sugar lovers include rats, horses, cows, sheep, goats, opossums and other marsupials, mice, and humans. Sugar haters include chickens, armadillos, hedgehogs, gulls, and cats. Cats are the obligate carnivore and cannot digest sugar. In contrast, humans like the taste of sweetness from infancy. It is fascinating to note that as a normal human eats more sucrose, the level of sucrase increases to enable digestion of the additional sucrose.

Sugar and Health

The disorders usually associated with ingestion of large quantities of sugar are dental caries, coronary heart disease, diabetes mellitus, hyperirritability, and obesity. We can quickly eliminate the misperceptions surrounding most of these problems. First, it has been said that if children eat too much sugar, it will increase their irritability. Further, it has been purported that some children are more sensitive to sugar than others. Neither of these conclusions has been substantiated scientifically. In fact, many studies have indicated that no relationship exists between the sugar intake of children and their level of irritability. Second, the amount of energy per gram of sugar is approximately four calories; the amount of energy per gram of fat is approximately nine calories. If you eat massive amounts of sugar, you will surely ingest large amounts of energy. Sugar alone, however, is not a cause of obesity. Obesity is generally a result of the ingestion of more energy than is expended, that is, too many calories are ingested for the number of calories that are expended.

Sugar also has been associated with diseases of the coronary arteries. In some people the ingestion of sugar increases triglycerides in the blood, a risk factor for coronary heart disease. In others, it does not, and the difference is probably genetic.

Dental caries is a major global public health problem. It is now becoming a problem in countries in which sugar was not consumed previously in large quantities. Caries is now prominent in Japan, for example, and it is a problem in Australia and the Philippines. Caries also exists where sugar is grown and children chew sugar cane. Consumption of sugar cane in Hawaii has caused a high incidence of caries. If infants or toddlers are permitted to keep bottles of sugar water in their mouths, their front teeth will decay. Caramels, toffees, and sugars that stick to the teeth are substances most likely to lead to caries. In malnourished children, caries can lead to systemic infection. Children who eat caramels or toffee should brush their teeth immediately afterward to remove the sugar from their teeth.

Diabetes mellitus is divided into two categories; insulin-dependent and non-insulin dependent. Insulin-dependent diabetes mellitus requires insulin and is found most often in children. Non-insulin-dependent diabetes is usually found in adults. Sugar is an important component in the diet of many persons with diabetes. Clinicians try to alter the diets of such patients by prescribing a reduction in the amount of dietary sucrose and an increase in the amount of complex starches, such as breads and pasta. The incidence of insulin-dependent diabetes mellitus is increasing dramatically. In an 80-year period in the United States, the incidence has increased from approximately five occurrences per 100,000 persons to 24 per 100,000. The incidence in France is approximately four per 100,000, but in Finland, it is approximately 34 per 100,000.

The influences on diabetes are both genetic and environmental. Non-insulin-dependent diabetes exists in a number of varieties. Worldwide, members of the Pima-Papago and the Apache tribes have the highest prevalence of the disease, followed closely by members of most other Native American tribes. By the age of 45, a Pima-

Papago has a 40% chance of having diabetes, and by 65, almost 70% of the women will have diabetes. Several theories exist to explain the presence of this type of hyperinsulinemic diabetes. One theory proposes that the stimulus for the development of diabetes in people with genetic predisposition is triggered by a change from a primitive diet to an industrialized diet. Kerin O'Dea studied 10 Australian aborigines who had diabetes. During the study they consumed their native high-protein, low-carbohydrate diet; the diabetes disappeared and they lost weight.

The basis for non-insulin-dependent diabetes is still not understood, but diet and sugar may be important. Today this type of diabetes is one of the more prevalent chronic diseases in the world. In the United States it occurs primarily among American Indians, blacks, and Hispanics. The incidence is increasing in Oceania and Australia. Peter Bennett suggests that if economic conditions improve and life expectancy increases in the developing nations, the prevailing trends will dramatically increase the worldwide incidence of diabetes.

The Eskimos had no sugar in their diet until about 50 to 100 years ago. Their diet was high in fat and protein and low in carbohydrate. (Incidentally, their cholesterol levels were low because of the unsaturated fatty acids from the cold-water fish and animals in their diet.) Among the Eskimos of Greenland and Canada, approximately one person out of five to ten is unable, because of genetic makeup, to digest sucrose. This phenomenon occurs in only one in 2000 of the non-Eskimo population.

Is there cause and effect between sugar consumption and diabetes? This question is the basis for many studies now in progress. The combined efforts last year of groups in Zurich and Boston to isolate the gene for sucrase will provide additional stimulus for the studies.

Most people can include sugar in their diet in moderation without health risks other than dental caries. Claims that sugar causes hyperirritability and obesity have not been substantiated. Diabetics and people with hypertriglyceridemia, however, must control their intake of sugar under the guidance of their physician.

Suggested Reading

Aykroyd WR. The story of sugar. Chicago: Quadrangle Books, 1967.

Gudmand-Hoyer E, Fenger HJ, Kern-Hansen P, Rorbaek Madsen P. Sucrase deficiency in Greenland: incidence and genetic aspects. Scand J Gastroenterol 1987;22:24-8.

Hamman RF, Bennett PH, Miller M. Incidence of diabetes among the Pima Indians. In: Levine R, Luft R, eds. Advances in Metabolic Disorders, Vol 9. New York: Academic Press, 1978:49-63.

Henning SJ, Kretchmer N. Development of intestinal function in mammals. Enzyme 1973;15:3-23.

Hobhouse N. Seeds of Change. New York: Harper & Row, 1987.

Hunziker W, Spiess M, Semenza G, Lodish HF. The sucrase-isomaltase complex: primary structure, membrane-orientation, and evolution of a stalked, intrinsic brush border protein. Cell 1986;46:227-34.

Newbrun E. Sugar and dental caries: a review of human studies. Science 1982;217:418-23.

O'Dea K. Marked improvement in carbohydrate and lipid metabolism in diabetic Australian aborigines after temporary reversion to traditional lifestyle. Diabetes 1984;33:596-603.

Schneider K. Did sugar get too good a deal? New York Times 1986(Nov 12):4.

Shafrir E. Effect of sucrose and fructose on carbohydrate and lipid metabolism and the resulting consequences. In: Beitner R, ed. Regulation of Carbohydrate Metabolism. Boca Raton, FL: CRC Press, 1985: 95-140.

West KM. Diabetes in American Indians. In: Levine R, Luft R, eds. Advances in Metabolic Disorders, Vol 9. New York: Academic Press, 1978:29-47.

Yudkin J. Levels of dietary sucrose in patients with occlusive atherosclerotic disease. Lancet 1963;1:1335.

Index

Milton Keynes UK
Ingram Content Group UK Ltd.
UKHW022109141024
449569UK00031B/1836

9 780824 785253